CLINICAL TOXICOLOGY
OF AGRICULTURAL CHEMICALS

Clinical Toxicology
of
Agricultural Chemicals

by

Sheldon L. Wagner, M.D.

Environmental Health Sciences Center
Oregon State University

NOYES DATA CORPORATION
Park Ridge, New Jersey, U.S.A.
1983

Library of Congress Catalog Card Number: 82-14421
ISBN: 0-8155-0930-8
Printed in the United States

Published in the United States of America by
Noyes Data Corporation
Mill Road, Park Ridge, New Jersey 07656

10 9 8 7 6 5 4 3 2 1

Library of Congress Cataloging in Publication Data

Wagner, Sheldon L.
    Clinical toxicology of agricultural chemicals.

    Includes bibliographies and index.
    1. Agricultural chemicals--Toxicology. 2. Agricul-
tural chemicals--Environmental aspects. I. Title.
[DNLM: 1. Chemistry, Agricultural. 2. Pesticides--
Adverse effects.   WA 240 W135c]
RA1270.A4W33 1983   615.9'02   82-14421
ISBN 0-8155-0930-8

Foreword

The clinical toxicology of agricultural chemicals and the environmental issues which have arisen as a result of the use of these chemicals are presented in this book. The subject is viewed from the social, economic, and scientific standpoints.

Agricultural chemicals—pesticides, herbicides, and other related chemicals—play a key role in maintaining the strength of the U.S. economy, since agriculture is a major U.S. industry and the U.S. is a prime exporter of food and foodstuffs. These facts underscore the continuing need for agricultural research. However, this need for new and effective chemicals must be balanced against the possible long-term detrimental effects to the environment. The issues are complex, and the book presents an overview of the problem, with the major thrust on scientific background and practical clinical toxicology.

The book is divided into two parts. Part I provides background information on the extensive use of agricultural chemicals and discusses some of the major environmental issues which have arisen as a result of their use. Understanding some of the basic concepts of this field may give the reader insight into the scope of the problems in determining possible genetic defects from exposure to any number of possible genetic insults, including chemicals. Laboratory methods and tests are described, and the role of regulatory agencies is discussed. Part II deals with the basic and clinical toxicology of selected agricultural chemicals, which have been classified according to chemical structure. Where possible, the discussion has included sections on basic chemistry, basic toxicology, molecular biology issues (teratogenicity, mutagenicity, carcinogenicity), environmental fate, potential human exposure, symptoms and signs of intoxication, and diagnosis and treatment.

The information in the book is from *Clinical Toxicology of Agricultural Chemicals* (PNRC Report 841-9) by Sheldon L. Wagner, M.D., of the Environmental Health Sciences Center, Oregon State University, prepared for the Pacific Northwest Regional Commission, August 1981.

The extensive table of contents provides easy access to the information contained in the book. An alphabetical list of the chemicals discussed is included, and the book is indexed.

Advanced composition and production methods developed by Noyes Data are employed to bring this durably bound book to you in a minimum of time. Special techniques are used to close the gap between "manuscript" and "completed book." In order to keep the price of the book to a reasonable level, it has been partially reproduced by photo-offset directly from the original report and the cost saving passed on to the reader. Due to this method of publishing, certain portions of the book may be less legible than desired.

Notice

This project was accomplished through funding provided by the Pacific Northwest Regional Commission. The statements, findings, conclusions, recommendations, and other data are solely those of the grantee-contractor, Environmental Health Sciences Center, Oregon State University and do not necessarily reflect the view of the Pacific Northwest Regional Commission. Funds for this publication were also provided by Oregon State University's Environmental Health Sciences Center through N.I.E.H.S. Grant ES 00210.

Preface

This book, written from a sense of perceived need, is offered in the hope that it will be useful to people of various interests and different training. Agricultural chemicals are a fact of life in this world and their universality has become controversial. There are many issues: social, economic, scientific and others. They are never addressed together yet the undertones of each are always present in any open meeting on any aspect of the subject. The issues, of course, are all complex but such complexity does not mean that they cannot, nor should not, be addressed even though the emotions may be intense and labile. It is hoped that this book will present a part of all aspects although it is not an in-depth analysis of each issue and the major thrust is the background and the practical clinical toxicology of these chemicals. For those interested in further reading, the chapters are followed by key references but are not meant to be complete bibliographies. Other sources of information are also listed. Although the book is written particularly for physicians, I believe that it should be useful to the understanding of various viewpoints by other disciplines and by the public at large. If such furthering of mutual understanding leading to increased communication occurs, the book will have, in my mind, achieved one of its major objectives.

Many thoughts and kind words of consideration are due to many people. I have learned much from many colleagues at Oregon State University, and in particular, I wish to thank Drs. Virgil Freed, Frank Dost and James Witt who have been, and always are, a great help in understanding this subject. I am also indebted to the following for their helpful review and comments on the rough draft of this material: Jack Allard, Eric Deck, Richard Ellerby, William Kosesan, Hershell Pendell, Nancy Stouffer, and Warren Westgarth.

Most significantly, I am indebted to, and this book would not have been possible without, the untiring efforts and enthusiasm of Carol McLaren. In addition to her multiple hours of hard work in helping at every level, her optimism, encouragement and even-keeled temperament will always be appreciated.

Sheldon L. Wagner, M.D.
Oregon State University
March 1981

Contents

Part II: Individual Chemicals

Part I
Scientific Background

Introduction

A common misconception held by the public is that the
United States' major strength in the field of industry is
related in some way to mechanization. The United States
is known historically as the founder of the industrial
and mechanical revolution and the conception of many people is that this reliance upon mechanics is the principal
source of economic strength in this country. The following statements made by Press (1978) may therefore be
rather surprising: 1) agriculture is this country's
largest industry, with assets of over $531 billion; 2)
the food and fiber industries are the nation's biggest
employers, with between 14 and 17 million people working
in some phase of them from growth to sales; 3) since
1971, U.S. agricultural exports have tripled to a record
$24 billion in 1977 resulting in a net contribution of
$10 billion to our balance of payments; 4) the United
States supplies about half of the grain that moves in
world trade and three-fourths of the soybeans. It produces about 70% of all the food aid to the world.

Conversely, again from Press, most nations in this
world are chronic importers of food and the situation is
growing worse. In 1950, some 45 nations exported food or
were self sufficient but by 1974, only 19 nations did so.
Only four countries, including the United States, accounted for more than 90% of the exports. The demand for
food in 80% of the entire Third World's population is in
excess of its supply.

These facts underscore the importance of agriculture
not only to this nation but to other nations of the
world. The need for continued agricultural research in
order to increase the yield of food available is of
major importance for the future. Agricultural chemicals,

3

including pest and weed control types, as well as other
related chemicals, play an important role in maintaining
the strength of this part of our economy. There is no
question that many of these chemicals have a significant
level of toxicity, particularly when applied or used incorrectly or inappropriately. Everyone is, therefore,
aware of the necessity of balancing the need for chemicals against the possible long-term detrimental effects
to our environment. The magnitude of assessing toxicity
of all chemicals is a continuing and impossible job. If
one recognizes that all chemicals are toxic given in inappropriate dose, route, and so on, then when one considers that there are now over four million known chemicals
with the number growing at approximately six thousand per
week and that there are now approximately 63 thousand
chemicals which are in common use, one can appreciate the
magnitude of the problem.

Recognizing that environmental factors probably play a
major role in the state of human health, the continued
surveillance and investigation into the relationship of
chemicals to health remains a major priority. A principal controversy with many agricultural chemicals has
been with respect to their long-term accumulation in the
environment, such as with DDT, and their potential as
possible agents to cause delayed health effects such as
birth defects, cancer, or genetic changes of future generations. We should recognize, however, that during the
past 25 years, certain diseases have decreased considerably in spite of, or perhaps because of, the introduction
of chemicals into our environment. For example, during
the past 25 years, heart disease, our major killer, has
decreased by more than 24%; stroke has dropped 32.5%;
deaths due to hardening of the arteries have decreased
53%. Other improvements could be cited. The above statistics are not meant to minimize the importance of chemically related health problems but simply cited to note
that a number of health parameters in addition to life
expectancy are continuing at this time to improve. Furthermore, many problems of health could be significantly
decreased if the public took on more of its own share of
responsibility in attempting to reduce actual self-in-
flicted diseases such as those associated with cigarette
smoking, alcohol, and other drugs.

Part I of this book is intended to provide readers
with information about the extensive and wide use of
agricultural chemicals and to discuss some of the major
environmental issues which have arisen as the result of

their use. Chapters in this section are directed at
basic pharmacology and toxicology to give readers a more
in-depth understanding of the scientific process. The
deeper the understanding of these basic disciplines, the
less superficial will be any approach to a discussion of
the environmental issues. Since the problems of birth
defects, ability to produce cancer, or other important
changes in our genetic make-up are frequently a major
point of discussion in the public eye, a section of
Part I is devoted to the field of molecular biology. It
is hoped that understanding some of the basic concepts of
this field will allow the reader to understand some of
the problems in determining the possible genetic effects
from exposure to any number of possible genetic insults,
including chemicals. The methods, and some of the problems, which are used to determine a significant genetic
change in laboratory tests are discussed. The methods,
and also the difficulties, in attempting to measure genetic changes in humans or in other parts of the actual
environment are also presented. These changes are particularly important in human beings in spite of the many
difficulties existing in measurement. Finally, the role
and importance of the regulatory agencies at all levels
of government can be confusing for anyone trying to decide where to seek information. The section on the regulatory agencies is intended only to give information on
the more important agencies in the Pacific Northwest and
federal government but is not intended to be all inclu-
sive. The role of the Environmental Protection Agency
and the regulation of chemicals via the RPAR process, in
particular, is addressed.

References

Press, F. (1978) Science and technology: the road
    ahead. Science 200:737-741.

1
Production and Uses
of Agricultural Chemicals

Determining the actual amount of agricultural chemicals used per annum is somewhat difficult to assess exactly. Figures are not available on an annual basis. Production figures are available. However, manufacture of chemicals may not be a reliable indicator of the actual usage in the United States since many chemicals are imported and exported. Usage patterns vary considerably by geographical location and season since crops vary from one region to another and the utilization of chemicals may also be dependent upon climactic variables. Time of the year and use of chemicals may vary since chemicals are not applied uniformly throughout the twelve months. A variety of governmental agencies may use chemicals in places not ordinarily expected or suspected. In general, surveys are attempted and are usually based upon a sample. These surveys usually are performed by government agencies, private firms under contract with the government, or private firms as a service performed for industry. Regardless of the method used, such surveys involve a considerable expense related to the difficulty of collecting complete data. Furthermore, the publication of the data commonly has a lag period which is several years behind the actual use. Surveys are performed in varying years by the United States Department of Agriculture. In 1974, the Council on Environmental Quality let a contract to the Midwest Research Institute for a use survey on data collected in 1972. The Doane Agricultural Service, located in St. Louis, Missouri, apparently performs an annual survey for manufacturers but this material is not readily available to the public since it represents a proprietary interest. New governmental regulations require industry to follow chemicals from manufacture to use or disposal.

The Agricultural Extension Department of the State of Washington performed a survey on the use of agricultural chemicals in farming for that state. A summary of that report follows.

In the United States, estimates of domestic consumption of pesticides have been made. The USDA in 1971, estimated that 833 million pounds were consumed. In 1972, the study for the CEQ estimated that 976 million pounds of material were consumed.

Use by Private Farmers - 1971

American farmers purchased fungicides, insecticides, herbicides, rodenticides, defoliants and desiccants, miticides, growth regulators, and other chemicals to use for production purposes. It is estimated that the application of agricultural chemicals by farmers account for about 60% of all domestic applications. The chemicals with the largest relative increase have been the herbicides which are now used frequently as a substitution for hand labor or machine cultivation. Sulfur is the most commonly used fungicide with 113 million pounds being used in 1971, which is approximately three times as much sulfur used as all other inorganic and organic fungicides. The common organic fungicides are the dithiocarbamates, compounds containing heavy metals such as iron (ferbam), zinc (zineb), or manganese (maneb). Other common organic fungicides are captan, chloranil and dichlone.

In the United States, the most commonly used herbicides are atrazine, 2,4-D, and propachlor. However, in the State of Washington, it is apparent that the most commonly used herbicide is 2,4-D and the most common crop to which herbicides are applied is wheat.

Insecticides are used regularly with approximately 90% consisting of synthetic organic chemicals. Since the cancellation of the use of DDT, the pattern of insecticide use has changed from the long-acting and potentially bio-accumulating chlorohydrocarbons to increased use of the more toxic organophosphorous materials, and the somewhat similarly acting carbamates. Generally, the use of insecticides is more concentrated on crops such as cotton and corn, leading to a marked geo-

INSECTICIDES

	Pears 21,000 Acres	Sweet Corn 31,270 Acres	Alfafa Seed 37,500 Acres	Potatoes 105,000 Acres	Hops 21,500 Acres	Apples 92,500 Acres	Wheat 2,720,000 Acres	Total Pounds Used
Perthane	40,000							40,000
Galecrom/Fundal	33,000							33,000
Guthion	22,801					245,386		268,187
Imidan	5,126							5,126
Parathion	2,577				12,487	328,613	12,148	355,825
Thiodan	5,695	286		189,000		164,202		359,183
Dimecron	167							167
Diazinon	1,668				36,025	268,095		305,788
Sevin		20,260				120,300		140,560
Lannate		21,847	93					21,940
Gurdona		190						190
Nudrin		20,475						20,475
Dimethoate			4,875				5,839	10,714
Trichlorton			56,200					56,200
Toxaphene			57,300					57,300
Demeton			6,463					6,463
Carbofuran			11,400					11,400
Phosdrin			4,000					4,000
Naled			15,814					15,814
Supracide			759					759
Malathion			580		13,437		25,000	39,017
Monitor				189,000				189,000

INSECTICIDES

	Pears 21,000 Acres	Sweet Corn 31,270 Acres	Alfafa Seed 37,500 Acres	Potatoes 105,000 Acres	Hops 21,500 Acres	Apples 92,500 Acres	Wheat 2,720,000 Acres	Total Pounds Used
Temik				157,000				157,000
Disyston				168,000			81,163	249,163
Thimet				52,500				52,500
Dibrom					1,000			1,000
Oxydemetonmethyl (Metasystox-R)			1,819					1,819
TEPP					33,300			33,300
Systox					538		1,750	2,288
Zolone						146,844		146,844
Phosphamidon						191,670		191,670
Dieldrin						70,850		70,850
Morestan						134,342		134,342
Superior Oil						472,188		472,188
Aldrin							26,084	26,084
Heptachlor							26,084	26,084
Disulfoton							1,178	1,178
Total/crop	111,034	63,058	159,303	755,500	97,147	2,142,490	179,246	

FUNGICIDES

	Pears 21,000 Acres	Sweet Corn 31,270 Acres	Alfafa Seed 37,500 Acres	Potatoes 105,000 Acres	Hops 21,500 Acres	Apples 92,500 Acres	Wheat 2,720,000 Acres	Total Pounds Used
Karathane	3,417					118,258		121,675
Copper Sulfate	10,251					11,400		21,651
Lime Sulfate	15,000					1,009,500		1,024,500 (Gal)
Sulfur Cmpds	27,336			63,000		13,680		104,016
Streptomycin	4,271							4,271
Dieldrin		133						133
Captan				945,000				945,000
Polyram				735,000				735,000
Difolatan				34,500				34,500
Maneb				33,600				33,600
Zineb					5,902			5,902
Manzate						327,000		327,000
HCB							25,509	25,509
PCNB							25,509	25,509
Total/crop	45,275 15,000 Gal	133		1,811,100	5,902	460,338 1,009,500 Gal	51,018	5,902 Gal

OTHER PESTICIDES (ACARICIDES, RODENTICIDES)

	Pears 21,000 Acres	Sweet Corn 31,270 Acres	Alfafa Seed 37,500 Acres	Potatoes 105,000 Acres	Hops 21,500 Acres	Apples 92,500 Acres	Wheat 2,720,000 Acres	Total Pounds Used
Plictran	1,424				96,508	98,068		196,000
Ethion	1,424					205,446		206,870
Omite	2,085		618		27,093	6,441		36,238
Endrin	2,085					4,275		6,360
Comite			6,205					6,205
Galecron			260					260
Kelthane			309		2,150			2,459
Azodrin				10,500				10,500
Tedion					1,075			1,075
Vendex						109,000		109,000
Total/crop	7,018		7,392	10,500	126,826	423,220		

HERBICIDES

	Pears 21,000 Acres	Sweet Corn 31,270 Acres	Alfafa Seed 37,500 Acres	Potatoes 105,000 Acres	Hops 21,500 Acres	Apples 92,500 Acres	Wheat 2,720,000 Acres	Total Pounds Used
Paraquat	6,834					22,800		29,634
Caseron	5,125					17,100		22,225
Simazine	1,822					6,080		7,902
Diuron	1,822					6,080		7,902
2,4-D	854	534				31,350	1,530,000	1,562,738
DNBP	1,500				9,450	5,700	12,500	29,150
Sinbar	2,001					10,640		12,641
Alachlor		25,155						25,155
Sutan		13,870						13,870
Atrazine		33,750						33,750
EPTC		12,000						12,000
Dinoseb		2,250						2,250
2,4-DB			900					900
Trifluralin			150	21,000	1,000			22,150
IPC			6,000					6,000
Eptam				63,000				63,000
Sencar				25,000				25,000
MCPA							306,000	306,000
Dicamba							102,000	102,000
Bromoxynil							102,000	102,000
Terbutryn							345,440	345,440

HERBICIDES

	Pears 21,000 Acres	Sweet Corn 31,270 Acres	Alfafa Seed 37,500 Acres	Potatoes 105,000 Acres	Hops 21,500 Acres	Apples 92,500 Acres	Wheat 2,720,000 Acres	Total Pounds Used
Linvron							95,200	95,200
Diallote							54,400	54,400
Barben							8,160	8,160
Chlorbromuron							31,008	31,008
Total/crop	19,958	87,559	7,050	109,000	10,450	99,750	2,586,708	

NEMATOCIDES

	Pears 21,000 Acres	Sweet Corn 31,270 Acres	Alfafa Seed 37,500 Acres	Potatoes 105,000 Acres	Hops 21,500 Acres	Apples 92,500 Acres	Wheat 2,720,000 Acres	Total Pounds Used
DD - Shell				1,050 Gal				1,050
Telone (Dichloropropane)				105,000 Gal				105,000 Gal
Temik				157,500				157,500
Total/crop				158,550 105,000 Gal				

graphic variation in the use of these materials. Nevertheless, considerable amounts are used on certain farm crops in the Pacific Northwest - particularly fruits and vegetables.

Other chemicals commonly used by farmers include the fungicides and fumigants, which are used to kill unwanted organisms in the soil and in storage buildings holding harvested commodities. Examples are the use of mixes of various chlorinated propanes or propenes and organic bromides. Defoliants or desiccants are not used commonly in the Pacific Northwest but are used extensively in the South in the harvesting of cotton in order to prevent a mixture of the cotton lint with the cotton leaves. Miticides, which are chemicals used to destroy mites and arthropod pests are used principally on fruit crops in the Pacific Northwest. The most commonly used miticide is probably chlorobenzilate.

Agricultural Chemical Use By Private Firms

A wide range of private commercial, industrial and institutional firms use a complex variety of pesticides in the direct conduct of their business and in the maintenance of their buildings or other facilities. Good data on use are not available although the use of these chemicals in these situations is generally considered to be "essential". That is, such usage probably allows a considerable economic advantage although data do not appear to be available for a precise analysis. Three major classes of firms using pesticides can be distinguished: firms providing pesticides as a service or retail product, firms producing a product requiring protection from pests, and firms providing a product that is aided by pesticides.

Firms Providing Pesticides as a Service

The provision of pesticides as a service is a specialized industry whereby these firms perform a service on a contractual basis to industry, to the public such as private homeowners, and to government agencies. Whether the actual measurement of the returns from this service received is enough benefit to society as a whole appears to be a major question nowadays. No general answer can be given to this question and it is suggested that appro-

priate assessment can only be done on a case-by-case
basis. Three different types of firms exist:

Pest Control Operators (PCOs): A PCO is a firm which
is engaged in selling its services to homeowners, commercial firms, industrial establishments, and non-profit
institutions, including governments. There are two major
types of PCOs - interior and exterior. The largest activity of interior PCOs is for termite control with the
most commonly used chemical being chlordane. Other commonly used chemicals are diazinon, dichlorvos and hepta-
chlor. Exterior PCOs are involved in a variety of vector
controls as well as control of unwanted plants and therefore chemicals used would include a variety of herbicides.

Custom Applicators: The term "custom applicators"
generally refers to those firms that specialize in selling their services to farms. Most material is applied
from fixed-wing aircraft with a lesser amount from a
variety of ground rig methods. Since aerial application
is common, one problem which does exist is that of potential drift outside of the sprayed area thus raising the
problem of application to undesired areas. When dealing
with chemicals which are clearly toxic, such applications are restricted by boundaries although the question
which is raised in terms of public health is the assessment of what constitutes safety and toxicity (see section on Safety). A significant hazard of aerial application occurs to the applicators themselves who are,
more than any other group, exposing themselves to significant health hazards secondary to their occupation.

Janitorial Supply Houses: This term simply refers to
those firms that are retail outlets for any variety of
agricultural chemicals for unrestricted use indoors.
Some commonly used chemicals are pyrethrin, a variety of
rat and mouse baits, etc.

Firms Producing a Product Requiring Direct Protection
From Pests

A wide variety of industries produce and market products which are subject to direct attack by various pest
organisms. These companies use pesticides as a step in
their manufacturing process in order to protect their
final product, i.e. to increase the yield, increase the

quality of the final product, stabilize production and
so forth. Examples of common industrial use for these
purposes follow:

Wood Processing and Manufacturing: The forestry industry is of major importance to the Pacific Northwest
states. The industry has a major economic impact but
also represents a significant environmental impact by
the very nature of the inate beauty of the living product. It is sometimes difficult for the public to understand that the lumber industry is in many ways quite
similar to farming excepting that the crop is harvested
every 50-100 years rather than annually. Both the production of the crop and the utilization of the product
occasionally demand the use of agricultural chemicals.
The following, because of its directness and simplicity,
is quoted from The National Academy of Sciences report
on Contemporary Pest Control Practices and Prospects
(1975).

> "The production of wood fiber from commer-
> cial forests is itself an industrial process
> utilizing pesticides. Once trees are harvest-
> ed, a new complex of pest organisms, including
> insects and fungi, threaten the timber prod-
> ucts. The specific nature of the pest problem
> depends upon whether the wood is destined for
> use as whole or nearly whole logs (such as
> utility poles or railroad crossties), lumber,
> or pulp and paper manufacturing.
> "A total of about 14 billion cubic feet of
> wood are removed from the American forest
> each year. A very small fraction of this to-
> tal (2%) is treated with preservatives. The
> value of the treated wood is estimated at
> about $450 million per year. The stake soci-
> ety has in the success of the preservation
> process, however, may be much higher than
> would be suggested by the volume and dollar
> value of the treated product. More than 50%
> of the treated wood is destined for service
> as railroad ties and utility poles, both of
> which play crucial roles in our transporta-
> tion and communication systems. Between 20-
> 25% of the wood is intended for use as lumber
> or timber and thus will play an important
> role in building programs.

"The vast majority of wood treated is
southern pine and Douglas fir. The location
of wood-preserving plants reflects the geographic distribution of these tree species,
and more plants are located in the Southeast
and the Pacific Northwest. Approximately 400
companies are in the industry; most are small
and privately owned, but four large corpora-
tions account for about 35% of the product
used.
    "Fungal sap stains constitute a special
problem in the lumber manufacturing. The
organisms produce a blue or brown stain that
results in loss of grade (and hence value)
of the lumber. The wood is dipped or sprayed
with pentachlorophenol compound as a control
measure. The value of the treated lumber is
approximately one billion dollars.
    "The production of paper and other wood
fiber products utilizes somewhat over one-
third of the harvested timber in the United
States. The wood is pulped in the process
under conditions favorable to the growth of
slimes consisting of fungi, bacteria, or
algae. Pesticides containing mercury were
at one time commonly used as slimicides in
paper manufacturing......but this purpose
declined steadily during the late 1960's
and in 1972 only 76 pounds of mercury were
so utilized. Such compounds as methylene-
bis-thiocyanate and organo-bromine compounds
have replaced the mercurial slimicides."

    In addition to the above, pentachlorophenol is a
pesticide commonly used as a wood preservative which is
rapidly replacing creosote. Other chemicals used in
smaller amounts as wood preservatives consist of heavy
metal complexes derived from arsenic, tin, zinc, and
copper.

Cotton and Other Textiles: Just as wood fibers are
subject to attack by various pests, similarly, a variety
of textiles, including cotton, are also subject to biodegradation and are, therefore, treated with rather similar chemicals.

Water: In situations where organizations must store
large amounts of water for use other than human consumption, this water must be protected from biodegradation
or changes in quality from unwanted organisms such as
weeds, algae, fungi, or bacteria. For this reason, a
variety of herbicides, algicides, fungicides, and insecticides are sometimes applied to water during storage or
transit. Furthermore, the control of mosquitoes as a
public health measure depends upon the use of insecticides.

Rights-of-Way: The control of vegetation along transportation corridors is considered extremely important.
Weeds along railroad tracks constitute a fire hazard,
shorten the life of railroad ties, reduce traction for
braking, reduce drainage, and foul the ballast. Some
attempts are made to do the work manually. Railroad
companies treat an estimated 1.6 million acres of land
with approximately 20 million pounds of chemicals each
year. The most commonly used materials are salts of
chlorate and borate, phenoxy herbicides, and bromacil.
Herbicides are also commonly used as part of highway
maintenance programs, partly to prevent weeds from
emerging through newly laid pavement but also to eliminate broad leaf plants in favor of grasses. The presence
of high grass along the roadsides may also constitute a
driving hazard. The transmission of electric power and
of telephone-telegraph communication depends, in part,
upon corridors for the wires and other devices. It is
particularly important that vegetation be prevented from
growing into, or falling upon, the transmission lines
and, therefore, these corridors are kept clear. The
principal chemicals used are the phenoxy herbicides.

Open Space: In many situations, particularly for
recreational purposes, open ground must be maintained.
The USDA currently estimates that there are about 20
million acres of such land across the nation, of which
3.8 million acres (19%) was treated with herbicides in
1968.

Agricultural Chemical Use By Government

Federal, State, and local governments are all involved in the use of agricultural chemicals in diverse
ways. Examples of such programs follow:

Programs Aiding Agriculture and Forestry: Two agencies of the United States Department of Agriculture
(USDA) - The Animal and Plant Health Inspection Service
(APHIS) and the Forest Service (FS) - have major programs involving agricultural chemicals and pest control
at the federal level. The APHIS activities include inspection, quarantine, and regulation designed to prevent
the introduction of pests into the United States and/or
to prevent the spread of pests beyond areas already in-
fested. Both chemical methods, such as pesticides, and
biological methods, such as sterile-male insects, are
utilized. Careful inspection of ports of entry is a
major program designed as an economic measure to prevent
pests from other countries from entering our country and
causing unexpected crop damage as well as being a significant public health measure. The size of this operation
is considerable and some indication can be derived from
the figures from 1971:

<u>Quarantine Inspections at Ports of Entry</u>

Airplanes	305,000
Vessels	53,000
Vehicles from Mexico	38,000,000
Baggage pieces	88,000,000
Mail and packages	64,000,000

In the above year, more than 21 million pieces of
cargo were treated to prevent the introduction of pests,
about a fourth of which was as a chemical treatment. In
addition to control at ports of entry, the APHIS also
conducts programs designed to prevent the spread of disease through interstate shipments of livestock or other
biologics.

The Forest Service conducts a wide variety of control
operations on large acreages of land. These operations,
on areas being used for reforestation, timber stand improvement, fire hazard reduction, and so forth, are designed to control pests as well as weeds.

Three agencies of the Department of the Interior -
The Bureau of Land Management (BLM), The U.S. Water and
Power Resources Service (formerly the Bureau of Reclamation), and The Bureau of Sports Fisheries and Wildlife
(BSFW) - also conduct a variety of operations using
chemicals. The BLM has the responsibility for 60% of
all federal lands, which comprises 20% of the nation's
total. Timber, livestock forage, wildlife habitat, and

public recreation facilities are all included and managed by the BLM. The U.S. Water and Power Resources
Service locates, constructs, operates, and maintains
facilities for the storage, diversion, and development
of water for the reclamation of arid and semi-arid lands
in the Western states. They conduct pest control operations for the control of weeds on irrigation facilities
such as irrigation canals serving in the area of ten
million acres (about 20% of the total irrigated area in
the Western states). The chlorophenoxy herbicides,
atrazine, dalapon, monuron, copper sulfate, acrolein,
and xylene, are among some of the commonly used chemicals.
The BSFW has responsibility for the use, perpetuation,
understanding, and enjoyment of sports fish and wildlife
resources. It conducts programs on the production and
distribution of hatchery fish, the operations of wildlife
refuges, regulation of migratory bird hunting, and the
management of fish and wildlife populations. Presently,
a rather controversial program is that of predator control, a major part of which is for the control of coyotes
and other predators in the Western states. The program
used compound 1080 (sodium fluoroacetate) or strychnine.
Predators are a serious problem on rangeland, particularly on small animals such as lambs.

Programs Controlling Disease: Rats and mosquitoes are
vectors for disease which are recognized for their public
health importance. Many programs are operated by local
health departments. Considerable variability exists from
area to area, depending upon local interest, need, and
annual budgets. Decreasing disease vector control has,
in some instances, been shown to increase incidence, e.g.
rodents and bubonic plague.

Programs For Recreational Purposes: A variety of federal, state, and local agencies, as well as private organizations, supply agricultural chemicals to improve
the recreational quality of an area. Assessment of the
cost-benefit relationship is very difficult to assess in
this situation and the "control" of such recreational
areas is sometimes very highly subjective in terms of
value to different individuals.

Programs For Military Purposes: History has recorded,
and been subjected to, a variety of major changes as the
result of the effects of pests and their role as vectors
of disease. Such diseases have been responsible for the

downfall of numerous armies and have, in this sense,
very clearly interferred with the conduct of war for
many centuries. Indeed, World War II was the first
major war in which disease among troops did not play a
significant role. The insecticide DDT was responsible.
In the Vietnam War, the Defense Department enlarged the
use of chemicals to include extensive spraying with herbicides of forest and crop land in South Vietnam. This,
almost from the beginning, has been a source of major
controversy and question. In South Vietnam, an estimated
3.58 million acres (8.6% of the country) was treated with
2,4-D, 2,4,5-T, picloram, and cacodylic acid. The political, ethical, and philosophical questions which arose
from this program continue to have an effect upon the use
of all agricultural chemicals.

Agricultural Chemical Use in the Home

The private citizen uses a considerable amount of
chemicals both inside and outside his home. The quantitative assessment of the amount used is very difficult
to determine although the size of the market is probably
significant. In 1970, the total retail value of all
pesticides sold in the United States was estimated at
$1,545 million, of which $298 million (19%) was in the
residential category. The actual percentage of pounds
of pesticides purchased and used by the citizen is probably considerably less than the 19% figure. The sale of
a unit of pesticide to the homeowner does not necessarily
mean that the package is completely used. That is, a
considerable amount is probably disposed of through the
garbage or by pouring into sewage systems. Regardless of
the amount used, for the average citizen, this use is
probably the point at which he encounters the highest
concentration of any agricultural chemical as opposed to
the incidental exposure encountered via the use by industry.
Not many studies on the home use of agricultural chemicals have been performed. In a study of the role of
social class and DDT pollution in Dade County, Florida,
significant correlations of DDT and DDE levels were demonstrated with social class, with higher levels being
found in the less affluent and the situation apparently
aggravated by conditions of overcrowding, inadequate fly
screening, garbage accumulation, and so forth. In part,
these problems had previously been somewhat managed by

the application of DDT. Since this chemical has been
banned, the implication is that human exposure to disease
vectors has been increased.

Another study performed in Southern Florida demonstrated that several pesticides which are most commonly
used in the garden could be detected in the air. In
Dade County, dichlofenthion and dursban were identified
in six different air samples collected on a monthly
basis in 1974. Diazinon was identified in four of six
collected samples. These findings were compared against,
and considered to be in striking contrast to, those observed in 1971 when air samples were taken in similar
localities within the Greater Miami area. In 1971, DDT
and its metabolites were regularly identified in the air
but were not identified in the 1973 and 1974 surveys.

Only one thorough survey has been performed on the
home use of pesticides in different cities: Lansing,
Michigan; Dallas, Texas; and Philadelphia, Pennsylvania;
and it was performed by the EPA. Slightly more than
750,000 pounds were used in the suburban areas of these
three cities in 1971 and homeowners used the bulk of the
material (609,000 pounds). This was broken down as
122,000 pounds of herbicides, 429,000 pounds of insecticides, and 69,000 pounds of fungicides. The major objective in the use of these chemicals was the improvement
of lawns and gardens. The most commonly used herbicide
was 2,4-D and the insecticides used in largest quantities
were chlordane, dicofol, dimethoate, and malathion. In
addition to the above quantitative findings, three other
conclusions were reached: first, the timing of applications in most residential areas is condensed primarily to
the last weeks of April and first weeks of May; second,
the rates of application on lawns are apt to be very
high compared to many agricultural uses with between five
and ten pounds of pesticide deposited per acre; third,
the homeowner faces such a complex variety of pesticides
when shopping that his choice is often based upon attrac-
tiveness of the packaging, familiarity with a trade name,
salesmanship, etc. versus the recommendations for use by
regulatory agencies. In addition, one might note that
many homeowners have no fear of the material and do not
carefully read the labels. In summary, the use of agricultural chemicals by private citizens does represent a
significant factor for exposure to the population.

References

National Research Council: <u>Pest Control: An Assessment of Present and Alternative Technologies; Volume 1: Contemporary Pest Control Practices and Prospects;</u> National Academy of Sciences, Washington, DC, 1975.

2

Background
of the Chemical Controversy

Most authorities would agree that the continued maintenance and development of the agriculture and forestry
industry is, at least in part, dependent upon the chemicals which we generally refer to as insecticides, herbicides, fungicides, etc. Similarly, control of disease
vectors and poisonous plants, as well as the management
of recreational and habitat resources, require the use of
these chemicals. Whereas the degree of such dependence
may vary in each particular situation, and, while the
necessity for alternative approaches to pest or plant
control by other methods needs to be continually investigated, it is clear that agricultural chemicals are presently a necessary and important part of our environment
if we wish to maintain the food and fiber level to which
we are geared. A clear understanding of the proper use
and the potential danger to human beings is required at
all levels from the general public to the research
scientist.

The safety practices employed in using agricultural
chemicals have come under heavy scrutiny from the public,
its elected representatives in government, and from a
variety of scientific disciplines. For example, a recent
report of the U.S. Senate Judiciary Committee states that
"regulation of agricultural chemicals is in a state of
chaos". In Oregon, the public has become sufficiently
aroused to enforce restrictions on the use of such chemicals as 2,4,5-T, restrict the spraying of roadsides with
2,4-D and 2,4,5-T, restrict the spraying of 2,4,5-T
around homes, develop new regulations on the use of
Thiram in forestry, and express concerns and questions

about the potential teratogenicity and carcinogenicity
of chemicals currently in use. Most often, public pressure leading to a government regulatory action rises out
of concern for the safety to human beings, not issues related to economics or questions of a basically scientific
nature. This book is therefore being written principally
to address the issues of human safety, but it must be
recognized that multiple disciplines are involved in
reaching this assessment.

Role of Multiple Disciplines

The safety of any chemical, whether man-made or natural, has traditionally come under the realm of toxicology.
The role of this scientific group is specifically to determine the adverse effects of chemicals not only upon
humans but on many living organisms. Indeed, the basic
thrust of the field is usually to perform studies on non-
humans and attempt to extrapolate this or to assess some
safety factor to humans based upon experimental studies
in lower forms. As will be explained in a later section,
this assessment is not always of a precise nature. And,
like any other science, scientific techniques change and
reassessment is a continuous process.

Major concerns for the safety of chemicals have been
expressed by scientists in the field of molecular biology. These concerns arise from a knowledge of the ability of chemicals to produce cancer (carcinogenesis) or to
produce changes in the genetic make-up of humans which
will be seen in future generations (mutagenesis). A
question which cannot be answered totally at this time,
is one of determining how much reliability can be placed
upon the existing techniques for the study and evaluation of either carcinogenesis or mutagenesis. That is,
are the techniques suitable for determining whether a
chemical is truly capable of producing a genetic change
and, if it is capable, can we reliably state that a
small amount of this chemical may be allowed in the environment? A further question is what are the final risks
society assumes?

Industry also has a great concern for safe practices
in the handling of chemicals. Hard economic pressures
arise, not only in the sense of monetary measure, but
also in the sense of providing the people of our nation,
and in some cases, of the world with the necessary food
and fiber. It also seems very likely that a future

phasis will be to develop educational programs for employees and users directed at the prevention of human disease which might occur from inappropriate use or handling of these chemicals. This will mean programs which are not only designed to prevent acute accidents but which will require education of employees relating to possible future hazards of chronic illness stemming from poor work practices. Industry is concerned with these problems but even the most concerned employer has difficulty in developing the needed information into some type of educational program.

In medicine, the average physician has very limited access to knowledge about the potential or real problems which are encountered with agricultural chemicals. The usual toxicology textbooks are either too brief or too broad in nature to deal with anything excepting clinical generalities about the various classes of compounds. The emphasis is on acute intoxication syndromes with very little discussion about the prevention or problems of chronic disease. Problems arise concerning the correct procedures to establish a diagnosis, the appropriate methods of laboratory analysis and the expected "normal" values, the interpretation of laboratory results, symptoms and signs resulting from a particular chemical exposure and specific treatment. These parameters are frequently unknown to the primary care physician, not necessarily out of a lack of interest, but because of the inability to find the material.

Although a considerable body of information on the clinical toxicology of agricultural chemicals does exist, it is widely scattered in a host of different journals which are most often of a non-medical nature, books and industrial or governmental reports. Moreover, much of it is not sufficiently well-organized to be of use to either the physician or others concerned with these chemicals.

Until recently, the physician's general lack of knowledge about agricultural chemicals has not been a very significant omission simply because the occurrence of any patient presenting in a physician's office with complaints which might be referable to agricultural chemicals was extremely rare. Recently however, perhaps because of the widespread publicity about these chemicals in the news media, more and more people are questioning whether there may be a relationship of their complaints to chemical exposure and are therefore asking for a clear-cut decision by the attending physician. This is not often an easy matter and frequently the best that

can be said is that an exposure-illness may possibly be
related in some cause and effect manner. Such statements
frequently only lead to further public concern which in
turn leads to political pressure and reactions by our
governmental regulatory agencies. The question then may
not be "is such public concern justified"? Obviously, if
people are told that they may have an illness which is
possibly related to a chemical exposure, the concern is
reasonable. Several responsibilities seem to be emerging. One is that the medical profession will need to become more sophisticated in its knowledge of toxicology
and toxic potentials as well as the correct symptomatol-
ogy related to environmental chemicals. Secondly, it may
be time for the public to become more aware that the medical profession is not necessarily a united front in ap-
proaching a disease process. Considering the hundreds of
medical schools in this country and the tens of thousands
of physicians, it is almost surprising that a good deal
of unanimity amongst the profession does exist. The
patients expect that the treatment of an acute appendici-
tis attack will not vary considerably from one physician
to another nor will the basic approach to the handling of
a patient with a chronic disease such as arteriosclerotic
heart disease or some chronic arthritic problem vary.
And indeed, this is the case. But, when one begins to
discuss preventive measures against disease, and this is
especially true of chronic disease, the cohesiveness of
opinion begins to disintegrate.

Commenting upon the difficulty of determining whether
tonsillectomies are necessary operations, a publication
by Carden (1978) states that even after extensive planning studies by a "blue-ribbon panel of experts", not
only could the procedure not be validated but the method
of studying the procedure could not be thoroughly agreed
upon. The author of the commentary then goes on to state
that,

> "It is difficult to explain such impotence
> to a public that has come to expect scienti-
> fic precision from medicine. Yet the inabil-
> ity to develop a study of unassailable scien-
> tific validity on an issue of such importance
> is testimony to the unique role the physician
> plays in the lives of his patients. Medicine
> is and apparently will continue to be an art
> based on science."

The above comments are also applicable to questions relating human health hazards to chemical exposure of the general society. In fact, the ability to develop studies of chemicals in human illness is far more difficult than that which could be developed for tonsillectomy studies since the population is not restricted and patients with tonsillectomies become part of a medical record system which can be searched retrospectively. Obviously the general population is not in any such system.

We are aware of the detrimental health effects from such habits as smoking, obesity, poor nutritional habits such as excessive carbohydrate or fat intake, the importance of sanitation and vector disease control and so forth. We cannot state, however, with precise assurance the exact importance of such parameters as psychological stress in developing a variety of organic syndromes of other bodily systems. In the case of chemicals, the exact relationship of any chemical exposure to the development of some future disease can be uncertain. Good estimates can be made and these are satisfactory to a large majority of clinicians. A group of people, whose devotees have certainly been audible in the Pacific Northwest, are willing to make much more precise statements concerning the fate of agricultural chemicals in the body. Since they may have a significant impact on the public in general, further discussion follows.

Human Ecology and Nutritional Therapy

These two fields, while not necessarily directly related scientifically, are a common focal point of arguments concerning the safety of chemicals in the environment. Although discussed separately, in practice, they are frequently entwined.

The field of "Human Ecology" or "Clinical Ecology" refers to a medical discipline which is practiced and/or investigated by a very small percentage of physicians. The term ecology is used straightforwardly in the sense of referring to the mutual relationship of organisms to each other. The use of the term human refers specifically to the effects of chemicals upon human beings in general and specifically refers to a clinically oriented investigational approach whereby the effects of chemicals can only be observed by first totally insulating an individual from his "total chemical environment" and then observing his response after re-exposure to parts of his chemical environment. The regime is clinically oriented because only symptoms are evaluated, i.e. patient complaints are not correlated with observable laboratory parameters. This makes the field highly subjective in nature, particularly in the production of acute symptoms. This approach is frequently referred to as "provocative testing". In addressing problems of acute illness, the approach is simply as described above, i.e. withdrawal and challenge. In the extension of chronic illness, the hypothesis states that chronic exposure to these chemicals results in chronic diseases which are traceable to the long-term exposure to chemicals, by an as yet unknown mechanism. The basic hypothesis states that the human being has evolved over the centuries via a system of adaptation which has taken thousands of years to develop; but, recent technological changes in our society have led to a plethora of chemicals to which the body can no longer correctly adapt. With the inability to "adapt", clinical symptoms then occur. It is not the purpose here to refute or agree with this clinical hypothesis. The field of "provocative testing" has been challenged editorially by more formal allergists with the request that scientific proof of this approach must be developed by the followers and not the disbelievers. The point to be made here is that once an individual is "diagnosed" as having a maladaptation syndrome to some type of environmental exposure, the individual is then necessarily required to avoid all exposure to the inciting agent regardless of dosage. If the inciting agent happens to be in an agricultural chemical, the difficulty of avoiding such exposure may become manifestly difficult in our present culture. For example, it makes little sense to grow organic gardens if the water used for irrigation is contaminated with a chemical which the patient believes to be the cause of personal illness. It is worthwhile to pause and note that in the field of Human Ecology, the dose-response curves seen in classic toxicology studies are not significant since the hypothesis states that any exposure, <u>regardless of dose</u>, will be detrimental. Since many members of the public are followers of this field because of personal beliefs related to health, it is perhaps not difficult to understand why emotionally charged and direct conflicts occur.

The field of "nutritional therapy" which is more commonly and rather patronizingly referred to as "food faddism" has a following which is probably far larger than is generally appreciated. In the context used herein, the term "nutritional therapy" refers to the use of such over-the-counter pharmaceuticals as vitamins, liver supplements vegetable extracts, trace mineral supplements, seafood tablets and so on. At the extreme end of this spectrum are those people who are devotees of "natural" foods, as opposed to the use of industrially processed foods. How widespread is nutritional therapy? There is no certain answer to this question but undoubtedly there are millions of followers in either a subtle or overt fashion. How many people take five to ten grams of vitamin C at the onset of a cold syndrome? How many millions of people take vitamin capsules on a fairly regular basis and thus help to support a multimillion dollar industry which, in fact, has little or no scientific basis? While it is quite appropriate for people to take vitamin tablets during recovery periods from certain kinds of stress, in the presence of particular types of acute or chronic disease or as a preventive measure against a chronically poor diet, most people take vitamin supplements in the hope of assisting their health status and not because of genuine vitamin deficiency. Moreover, a certain percentage of people take vitamin tablets daily because they instinctively feel that their health is improved or that they "feel better" by such daily supplementation. As stated, this practice is certainly widespread. One need only walk into any local pharmacy and peruse the shelves of vitamin supplements which are readily available and regularly sold in order to get some concept of the magnitude of this established behavior pattern. While the aforementioned practice represents a subtle form of nutritional therapy, at the other extreme is the use of megavitamin dosages, the food supplements and so on. Most physicians have no concern over the frequency of this practice simply because the use of vitamins, whether in usual replacement dosages or in megavitamin therapy, is, with the exception of vitamin A and vitamin D, no hazard. Excessive amounts of other vitamins are usually excreted without leading to human toxicity.

For the natural food devotee, there is an obvious conflict between the use of synthetic chemicals in the environment and the individual's right to practice his personal nutritional philosophy. The use of chemicals then becomes a matter of invasion of personal privacy as much as, and perhaps more than, any other issue. The argument against "food additives" is frequently based upon bonafide scientific experiments in animals or observations in human beings in which, as in Human Ecology, an attempt is made to extrapolate between high dosage results and the very low end of the scale in which low dosage may or may not be considered harmful.

One should not conclude from the above that it is only the human ecologists or nutritional therapy followers who have a health interest at stake in the use of chemicals in our society. However, it is reasonable, when one hears a question about the health effects of some environmental chemical to also question the individual or group about the specific reasons for their health concerns. To correctly identify these groups of people would undoubtedly lead to considerably fewer arguments and would at least place many of the questions relating to human health effects and environmental chemicals in the proper frame of reference.

Role of the Press

The role of informational media - radio, television, and newspapers - is one of major importance in the public's understanding of the problems and tentative solutions to the use of agricultural chemicals. Whereas problems seemingly are easily identified, actually the definition of a problem in the eyes of the public needs to be more clearly defined and the news media, in particular, needs to have an understanding of when a problem truly exists or is demonstrated to exist rather than when a problem is merely implied.

This important distinction is not easily clarified by scientific writers without a major effort. The scientific process frequently leads to a situation where more questions are raised than are answered. Scientists are under heavy scrutiny from peer review prior to acceptance of experimental studies and publication in any scientific journal. When experimental results are given to the press and to the public without the peer review process, the possibility of gross misinterpretation is not unlikely. Although it is extremely difficult for scientific writers to find the time to understand the complexities of any single problem, it would seem that such understanding is vital in order to correctly inform the public.

Scientific Responsibility

The news reporter is not the only guilty party in this type of misinformation. The scientist also holds a responsibility to let reporters know that information being given to the public may be controversial. If the reporter becomes more informed about the scientific process, the less likely he is to fall into the trap of reporting information which is not acceptable to the large majority of scientists.

The tentative nature of science is not frequently understood nor is that of the tentative nature of the regulatory process which governs the use of agricultural chemicals. The public needs to understand that the regulatory process is a flexible one and that as scientists develop new information, the regulatory process changes in accordance with new information. The public has begun to believe that scientists can evaluate a chemical and state with absolute certainty that such chemical is totally safe. In fact, the scientific process allows only for the understanding that a chemical has a relatively low risk or that it is relatively safe at levels to which the public is being exposed. The public needs to be educated to the fact that our scientific understanding of chemicals is hindered by a good deal of uncertainty which will only change with time. The temporal nature of the process of accumulating new and discarding old ideas will lead to changes in society's acceptance of what is or is not safe. The press, if it has a major role, must educate the public to this type of thinking. In particular, it must eliminate the reporting of scientific problems as facts for which there is little argument.

This is not to say that the press should not report incidences of any nature which the public might perceive to be a problem. It does seem important, however, that the public's information about health be presented as developing questions and not necessarily as existing problems.

The importance of the public in determining the regulatory process is often not appreciated. The regulatory process responds to pressure from the public. When the public is misinformed, such regulatory processes may become more a matter of emotion or pressure from organized groups rather than regulation based upon scientific understanding. The subject is further discussed by Burger (1972).

Safety

The question repeatedly put to scientists, and always
with an answer expected, is: "Is this chemical safe?"
Unfortunately, the answer is not an easy one. Worse, the
meaning and interpretation of "safety" is interpreted
incorrectly. We have begun to assume that a safe chemical is one without any hazard, whereas no such chemical
truly exists. According to Lowrance (1976), it is time
to make everyone aware that "safety" is a term best defined as a state where the risks involved are acceptable
to society. Thus the term is relative and not absolute.
What is safe today to our society may be judged differently in another time or culture. Several centuries ago
man would have been considered insane to even consider
flying whereas nothing whatsoever was thought of dumping
raw garbage into city streets. In the future, our progeny will doubtless look upon many of our present-day
practices as foolhardy or naive. Thus "safety" is relative and also flexible. Furthermore, having defined
safety as an "acceptable risk", how does one determine
what the risks really are and who shall make the judgement of something being acceptable?

The role of determining risk of chemical exposure has
been an accepted procedure of the scientist: toxicologist, chemist, biologist, veterinarian, physician and
so on. The scientist can only describe risks but he cannot truly decide if such findings are acceptable to society, i.e. safe. In deciding when a risk is or is not
acceptable, the final decision is made by the public and
its regulatory agencies. This is a far from perfect
system but it is the system we use. In passing judgements of safety, we should recognize that two distinctly
different inputs exist - the public and the scientific.
Both parties have certain roles as well as responsibilities. When an issue of safety becomes emotional, individual roles and responsibilities sometimes get entangled
or lost.

On the other hand, the scientist (or the skilled tech-
nician) has every right to express individually perceived
concerns to the public. Assessing the importance of such
concerns is where the public is liable to become confused.
The late Sir Bertrand Russell made the following statement which still holds true.

"...Provinces of Knowledge border on a cir-
cumambient area of the unknown. As one comes

into the border regions....one passes from
science into the field of speculation."

It is important for everyone to recognize the above tru-
ism, although the implication is a bit subtle. Expressed
differently, Russell said that if any scientist asks
enough questions, a point is reached where answers given
are theoretical and open to question or debate. The
responsible scientist or technical authority is aware
when known facts come into the arena of conjecture - and
should say so to the public. The individual in a position of authority based upon knowledge is freely pros-
tituting himself when an advocacy position is taken and
statements are dogmatically made to the public which are,
in fact, in the "border regions", i.e. open to considerable scientific or technological debate and question. In
the emotional arena of safety of chemicals in the environment, scientists should state the known facts. When
extrapolation or personal judgements are made, they
should be stated as personal opinion and the public
should be aware of their personal nature. As cited by
Lowrance (1976), the role of the scientist was summarized by Rabinowitch.

"In adversary proceedings in which science
or one of its applications (such as technology, medicine or psychiatry) are involved,
both sides enlist the cooperation of experts -
scientists for the prosecution and scientists
for the opposition. This procedure makes a
mockery of science; in fact, it often comes
dangerously close to its prostitution.
"Juries, parliaments and electorates,
when called upon to judge between contesting
claims, often are unable to judge the arguments of their scientific experts rationally,
and often rely on the impression the competing
experts make on them, on their formal creden-
tials, and on the forensic quality and vigor
of their presentation.
"In the controversy over nuclear bomb
tests, some scientists, called upon by opponents of testing, emphasized the absolute
number of radiation-induced bone cancers
and leukemias likely to be caused by continued testing in the atmosphere; while
other scientists, called upon by advocates

of testing, stressed the low number of
expected victims, compared to the general
incidence of these malignancies. The first
group of scientists used the data to claim
that continued testing in the atmosphere
would be criminal, while the second group
used the data to argue that there is no
reason to discontinue the tests. Laymen,
including legislators, concluded that one
cannot trust scientists: some of them say,
'Stop tests - they are too dangerous';
others, 'Go on, you will not notice the
difference'. Yet, as scientists, the adversary experts did not disagree on the
facts of the situation; they disagreed only
on moral conclusions which they derived
from these facts - a disagreement in which
the judgement of scientists is no more,
while no less, valid than that of any other
citizen cognizant of the facts.

"Scientific experts called upon in liti-
gation or in political controversies should
not be used as partisan assistants in the
adversary process, but as impartial investigators to provide an agreed upon summary
of the relevant facts as well as the logical derivations from these facts. If needed,
the summary should clearly present differing
interpretations of the scientific evidence
and differing moral or political presumptions leading to different practical conclusions...

"Scientists, psychiatrists, physicians
and technologists should be asked to analyze
a problem, and to render their conclusions,
without advance presumption as to what
point of view they are to defend. If,
at a certain point, their conclusions begin
to be affected by extra-scientific reasons,
they must have sufficient intellectual
honesty to state: 'Up to this point, I
spoke as a scientist; from here on I will
speak also as a politically, ethically or
ideologically committed citizen...'.

"Scientists will not always be able to
make this distinction clearly; but, at
least society must not encourage them to

behave unscientifically, to conceal their
bias, or to resort to untruth or suppression
of a part of evidence."

What is the responsibility of the public and its regulatory agencies who make the final decision of acceptable
risk? Again, it is time to realize that safety does not
imply no hazard whatsoever. When a person drives an
automobile, each year a risk of death from accident is
taken (rather casually) of one in every 4,000 people.
The benefits of driving are so obvious and so necessary
that no one raises the issue of removing all automobiles
from the country and the well-documented risk is acceptable. In the case of agricultural chemicals, the benefits are not so easily seen but the risk, e.g. death or
disease, may be no greater. Before decisions of accept-
ability are made, the public should know as precisely as
possible what risks are known and what risks are conjectural. In order to find these answers, they must specifically ask authorities into which category the risk
falls and not, as is often the case, accept all statements as fact and assume only that differences of opinion
exist. These differences of opinion are the border
regions to which Russell refers. They must be recognized
as such! We should also realize that there will always
be grey zones and that answers to questions within those
areas are to be found at some future time.

The responsibility of regulatory agencies is huge -
nearly monumental at times. They must not only assess
risks but are required to make a judgement of risk versus
benefit; they must accept the will of the public and its
representatives. In the former case, benefit is an ag-
glomeration of economics and society's attitudes. Figures on economic gain or loss can be supplied by industry.
Societal attitudes are often more subjective. The public
will organize into advocacy groups as a means of being
more effectively heard. Such groups, when involved in
the regulatory process, should be questioned about their
fundamental philosophy, their numbers, their geographic
area of representation and other demographic variables.
To use the old axiom that the squeaky wheel gets oiled is
not a very satisfactory method of solving problems which
affect all society. The above is also inherently true
for industry.

What responsibilities to safety are held by the employer and employee? The chemical manufacturer holds the
responsibility of pre-marketing testing - already spelled

out by regulatory process – and safe and reliable production. The applicator should be held responsible for
proper application and the education of his employees
regarding not only safe working procedures but potential
hazards or concerns of the public. Both employee and
employer working with chemicals must accept the fact that
any chemical entails some degree of risk. These risks,
when given to the employee in full disclosure, should be
an accepted part of the job. That is, employees who
refuse to follow outlined safety procedures – for whatever
personal reason – should not be further employed in that
particular position. The employee must accept responsibility to his employer, to the public and to himself.

Finally, everyone should remember that the development
of safety regulations is not rigid, but is a flexible,
on-going process, as expressed in the HEW Report of the
Secretary's Commission on Pesticides (1969).

> "In weighing potential health risks against
> potential benefits it must never be forgotten
> that even the most far-seeing view may be
> proved erroneous by unexpected new scientific
> developments or by an altered attribution
> of those risks considered to be of utmost
> importance. An instance may be cited in
> the area of non-nutritive sweeteners. Ear-
> lier safety evaluations took into account
> softening of stools as the likely risk
> presented by high intake of cyclamates.
> Now one source of concern is the possibility
> of carcinogenesis brought about by these
> products or materials derived from them.
> Thus safety evaluation is an edifice whose
> construction is never completed; nor does
> it remain functional without periodic recon-
> struction. Strangely enough, both regulatory
> agencies and the public view as loss of face
> the frank recognition that many earlier
> decisions on safety must inevitably be
> proved wrong as scientific knowledge grows.
> There is nothing absolute about such decisions.
> All that we have a right to expect at the
> time they are made is that they should be
> the products of scientific competence and
> experience, mature judgement and full pos-
> session of all existing data."

References

Burger, E.J. (1972) Perspective on...public information, science, and the regulatory process. Environ Health Perspect 5:1-3.

Carden, T.S. (1978) Tonsillectomy - trials and tribulations. JAMA 240:1961-1962.

Lowell, F.C. (1975) Some untested diagnostic and therapeutic procedures in clinical allergy. J Allergy Clin Immunol 56:168-169.

Lowrance, W.W. (1976) Of Acceptable Risk, William Kaufmann, Inc., Los Altos, CA.

Randolph, T.G. (1976) Human Ecology and Susceptibility to the Chemical Environment, Charles C. Thomas, Springfield, IL. Fifth Printing.

Randolph, T.G. (1977) Both allergy and clinical ecology are needed. Ann Allergy 39:215-216.

Rea, W.J. (1977) Environmentally triggered small vessel vasculitis. Ann Allergy 38:245-251.

USDHEW (1969) Report of the Secretary's Commission on Pesticides and Their Relationship to Environmental Health, U.S. Government Printing Office, Washington, DC.

3

Toxicology

Introduction

The term "toxicology" is a word and a scientific
field which is presently widely used and abused. This
scientific discipline, which is a branch of pharmacology,
probably had as it's raison d'etre the study of injurious
effects of chemicals upon living organisms. In the past,
its principal association, and perhaps its principal use,
was to study incidental or criminal poisoning which
occurred as the result of some chemical response. The
field thus has a strong connotation with the use of the
lay term "poison". In fact, the medical dictionaries
still define toxicology as the science of the study of
poisons. Today, however, this is a very simplistic and
narrow definition which is no longer acceptable because
the unfortunate connotation is very deleterious. The
role of the toxicologist today is to scientifically
assess the risks each of us encounters in our ubiquitous-
ly chemical society. Current emphasis is not only upon
the role of chemical interaction with man, but also upon
the effect of chemicals on the environment, including the
entire biosphere. In our present society with its multiple problems ranging from overpopulation on the planet
surface to the greenhouse effect from increased carbon
dioxide levels at the outer surface of our atmosphere,
the toxicologist is now being called upon to actively
assess the manner in which man coexists with his entire
environment. The pressures are huge since in one case
injurious effects to the environment are undesired by
everybody and in the other, the beneficial effects of

chemicals cannot simply be overlooked. If present and
future generations wish to "return to nature", it is
important that this be a voluntary choice and not one
which is forced upon humans by one of the four horsemen.

Toxicology will be defined in this text as the study
of injurious effects of chemical substances upon any
living organisms. This is to distinguish it from physical interactions and to take it clearly out of the realm
of "arsenic and old lace". The field not only embraces
the study of chemicals upon the body but also the study
of the body upon chemicals. An understanding of this
scientific discipline is critical to discussion in this
text of any pathological processes encountered from
agricultural chemicals.

Mechanism of Drug Action

Given any drug, whether beneficial or toxic effects
are being evaluated, a lengthy and complex series of
steps must occur prior to any biological response. Even
the dose is not an absolute measurement since the drug
effect is not only dose dependent but is also form dependent. That is, a one gram unit of a chemical which is in
a single solid mass is far less likely to have any particular effect than the same gram which has been disper-
sed into millions of particles with each particle capable of leading to some future effect. The series of
events leading to a particular action is divided into
three specific phases. These are generally referred to
as the pharmaceutical phase, the pharmacokinetic phase,
and the pharmacodynamic phase. In toxicology, the corresponding phases are referred to as the exposure phase,
the toxokinetic phase, and the toxodynamic phase.

Exposure Phase

Given a chemical in the environment - a "dose" - the
presence of that chemical does not always mean exposure
in the toxicological sense. It is simply not enough to
state that because a chemical is present and humans may
also be present that some type of cause and effect relationship of beneficial or detrimental nature may occur.
For exposure to have a significant biological action, a
route of absorption must be supplied and available. Furthermore, it is important for the clinician to not only

determine the chemical but also determine the duration
that the individual has been exposed, the concentration
at which the chemical was present and then the route of
exposure. There are three routes by which any drug can
get into the body: the dermal (skin), the gastrointestinal system or the respiratory system. In occupational
medicine, the skin and respiratory routes are the most
important measures to be assessed. In the context of
environmental medicine and incidental exposure, the
gastrointestinal tract takes on more significance. That
is, the ability of some chemicals to move through the
food chain and finally become ingested is an issue whose
importance is widely debated.

The skin is a barrier of considerable magnitude in
its capability of protecting the human from exposure.
However, there are a number of variables which can break
this barrier down and which need to be taken into consideration when assessing possible chemical exposure. In
general, the skin is very resistant to the absorption of
water soluble chemicals, assuming that the chemical itself is non-caustic and by prolonged exposure will not
injure the epidermis. (One can get very cold in a heavy
rain shower or a swimming pool but the body will not
absorb any water.) Any dermatological disease will, on
the other hand, immediately provide an opening for chemical entry and should always be considered significant.
People with chronic skin diseases should not be working
in potentially toxic environments as open cuts or abra-
sions present an easy entry source for otherwise impermeable chemicals. The skin will, however, absorb fat
soluble chemicals without too much difficulty, regardless
of the condition of the epidermis. Thus, the nature of
the chemical itself is significant in considering exposure problems. Heat may play a role since as people
sweat, dusty chemicals which would normally not be
absorbed may become dissolved and, therefore, may be
absorbed. Clothing or other protective measures will
obviously prevent skin absorption providing the clothing
itself is cared for and properly laundered.

The respiratory tract, particularly the lung, represents an easy point of entry for chemicals which are in
the form of a gas or are aerosol. It is important to
distinguish between an aerosol and a particulate since
particulate matter does not get absorbed into the terminal part of the airway and is generally much less dangerous than aerosols. As a general rule, particulate matter
can be seen - such as smoke - whereas aerosols tend to be

invisible excepting in high concentrations. Movement
of chemicals into the terminal lung does not necessarily
mean that dangerous absorption has occurred. Again, the
nature of the chemical is important and certain chemicals
may simply stay in the lung for years without significant
impingement upon lung function. Finally, the respiratory
rate of an individual is important in determining exposure via the respiratory route. The worker who is breath-
ing heavily from exertion will obviously absorb considerably more chemical because of the increased respiratory
rate than will the individual at rest.

Toxokinetic Phase

Following exposure, the toxokinetic phase, also called
the pharmacokinetic phase, occurs. During this phase,
the chemical leaves the external environment and the
processes of absorption, distribution, metabolism and
excretion occur. These processes do not occur in any
random fashion but follow well studied and predictable
routes of biological actions.

The processes of absorption, distribution, and excretion occur by one or both of two methods - active transport or passive transport. The simplest, passive transport, refers to the diffusion of a chemical across a
membrane which is entirely dependent upon the difference
in concentration on both sides of the membrane. This is
defined as the concentration gradient. The ease with
which the substances diffuse across the membrane, called
the diffusion constant, determines the rate of passage.
The diffusion constant is dependent upon such factors as
the thickness of the membrane - chemicals absorb with
more ease across a mucous membrane than the skin; the
basic properties of the chemical; and the concentration
gradient itself. If the material is quickly distributed
away from the point of entry such that the concentration
gradient remains the same, one can graph a straight line
relationship between the rate of diffusion and the concentration gradient. This is illustrated in Figure 1.

The second method of transport, active, is a system
whereby the body actually requires energy and thus represents an active metabolic process of the body. The
active transport systems are much more complicated.
Chemicals will interfere with one another as they compete
for transport. Some chemicals are "preferred" because of
a selectivity phenomenon of some type of transport mech-

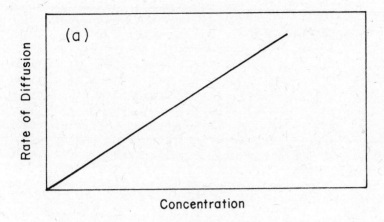

Figure 1

anism. Most transport systems prefer compounds which
are water soluble as opposed to fat soluble. Large molecules, such as proteins, cannot directly cross membranes
at all but rather are absorbed through a process called
pinocytosis whereby the cell membrane actually circum-
scribes the protein and then the entire membrane and
protein is pulled into the interior of the cell where the
protein is then released. The point to be made is that
transport processes are rate limited. Increasing the
concentration does not increase the amount of absorption
as in the case of simple diffusion but instead a maximum
amount of absorption is reached which is dependent upon
the mechanism of carriage across a membrane wall or via
some carriage system in the blood or other tissue. This
process is illustrated in Figure 2.

Before one can even consider the mechanisms of the
toxokinetic phase, one must first approach the chemistry
of the compound under scrutiny since such processes as
absorption, distribution and excretion are not only
dependent upon body mechanisms but are also dependent
upon the basic chemical structure of any compound. Most
important is the distinction between hydrophilic and
lipophilic substances. Simply expressed, hydrophilic
compounds are those that prefer to be dissolved in water.
Lipophilic compounds are substances which prefer to be
dissolved in fat or an organic solvent, such as chloroform. The capabilities of compounds that dissolve in
either water or an organic solvent can be expressed

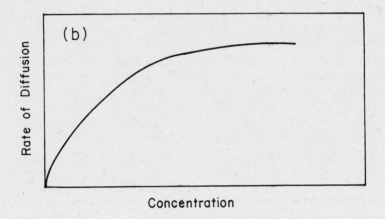

Figure 2

precisely in terms of the partition coefficient, the
relative concentration of the division of a substance
over two phases (water phase versus organic phase). A
partition coefficient is an important measurement of
chemicals, not only in the human body, but also how it
moves through the environment. Examples of hydrophilic
chemicals are strong acids, strong bases, and organic
compounds that have many free OH groups. In general,
hydrophilic compounds tend to be easily ionized. Examples of highly lipophilic compounds are organic solvents
in which there is very little free charge and no free
hydroxyl or other ionic groups available, such as benzene, octane and nitrobenzene. There is also a class of
organic compounds referred to as surfactants in which
half of the molecule is lipophilic and the other half is
hydrophilic. These compounds have strong detergent
properties and thereby have the capability of breaking
apart more complex organic compounds for more ease in
absorption. Another important property of chemicals
during the toxokinetic phase is the ability to bind
protein and, therefore, be transported or possibly inactivated. Since this is a competitive action, one
compound may actually remove another one in the process
of binding to a blood protein carrier - the albumin.
In summary, while exposure may occur, a chemical may,
in fact, not ever be absorbed because of its nature.
A very mildly lipophilic or hydrophilic compound is
unlikely to be absorbed through the gastrointestinal
tract. In contrast, highly hydrophilic or highly lipo-

philic compounds will move very quickly across internal
barriers. The presence of a natural surfactant, such as
human bile, will improve absorption. The internal pH,
i.e. the acidity or alkalinity, will result in a chemical
being ionized or not ionized as it enters the body. If
the chemical is in the ionized form, it is more likely
to be absorbed - or possibly excreted. Therefore, a
chemical already in the body can have marked changes in
excretion simply by changing the pH of the urine to
allow for ionization of the chemical and excretion
through the kidneys.

Given that a chemical has been absorbed and is being
transported or has been transported to a possibly active
site, a number of biochemical alterations can occur.
These biochemical alterations generally "detoxify" chemicals although in some cases the biotransformation process may actually result in increased toxicity. These
changes are important for a toxicologist to determine
since they represent the full understanding of the process by which any chemical works. Two types of biochemical alterations are known to occur and they are categor-
ized into either degradation reactions or conjugation
reactions.

The most important degradation reactions occurring
are hydrolysis, oxidative degradation, and reduction.
By hydrolysis one refers to the splitting of a compound
in two parts such that to one part a hydroxyl group (OH)
is added and to the other part hydrogen (H) is added. A
common example of this type of reaction is the degradation of an ester into an alcohol and an acid. The
process proceeds by an enzyme mechanism. If the ester
is highly resistive and also is lipophilic, it tends to
accumulate in fat tissues of the body rather than being
prepared for excretion by hydrolysis. The esterase
enzymes are present at high levels in the plasma, liver
and central nervous system. Certain agricultural chemicals, such as the organophosphate type, use as their
mechanism of action the ability to inhibit normally
occurring esterases, in this case cholinesterase. Since
most insects have a very low level of cholinesterase as
compared to mammals, the compounds can selectively kill
insects whereas the same level of organophosphate in the
mammal will have no significant effect. Conversely,
treatment of organophosphate intoxication is dependent
upon reactivation of the cholinesterase enzyme using
oxane chemicals. This class of chemicals is very effective in reversing the toxic effects of organophos-

phates. The pharmacological problem is that the oxanes
do not cross the blood brain barrier and, therefore,
will not reverse organophosphate intoxication of the
central nervous system.

A second type of degradation action is referred to as
oxidation which, as the term implies, is the use of an
enzyme to add oxygen to any foreign substance. This
process occurs principally in the liver and, particularly, in the plasmic reticulum. Oxidation may occur directly to a relatively free oxygen group, such as seen
in alcohols or aldehydes. In the case of long chain
organic compounds, the oxidation generally occurs in a
chain-step mechanism in which two molecules of carbon
are repetitively split off of the carbon chain. The
process of oxidation is important in nature as a natural
degradation mechanism, In general, oxidation will occur
on unbranched carbon chains but has more difficulty
occurring when a branched molecule is present.

Reduction is the least common of all types of degradation reactions. An example would be reduction of a
dithio compound such as $R-S-S-R^1$ being reduced to the
two compounds RSH and R^1SH. In general, degradation
reactions decrease the size of the molecule which increases their hydrophilic nature and also increases
their electric polarity because of the increased availability of the OH groups, NH_2 groups, and COOH groups.
These groups are then suitable for the other major type
of biochemical reaction - conjugation reactions.

Conjugation reactions are defined as the introduction
or addition of another molecule to an existing chemical.
This molecule usually is strongly acid in nature, examples being conjugations with glucuronic acid, amino
acids, sulfuric acid, and acetic acid. The conjugation
markedly increases the original chemical's hydrophilic
nature and, therefore, allows it to be much more rapidly
excreted. Alcohols seem to prefer to conjugate with
glucuronic acid. Carboxylic acids prefer to conjugate
with glycine. Phenols seem to especially prefer conjugation with sulfates (thus pentachlorophenol exposure and
absorption can be measured by the phenol-sulfate byprod-
uct excreted in the urine). Other examples of conjugation are methylation, the addition of a CH_3 molecule;
acetylation, the addition of an acetic acid to amino
group; and chelate formation, the addition of a heavy
metal ion to another chemical thereby detoxifying the
heavy metal.

Excretion Versus Retention

Excretion of chemicals occurs through the skin via the sweat glands, through the lungs via expiration, through the gastrointestinal tract and through the kidneys. In the case of the gastrointestinal tract, when chemicals are absorbed into the liver and then transported out of the biliary system into the upper gastrointestinal tract, these chemicals may temporarily be recycled through the enterohepatic circulation. Regardless of the route, excretion does follow the same set of rules, i.e. active or passive transport, utilized in absorption and distribution. Furthermore, excretion rates can be calculated from experimental data and such rates will take on a recognized and reproducible graphic form. Compounds which are highly hydrophilic or are themselves converted into water-soluble metabolites generally are kept in the body for only a very short period of time, whereas those compounds which are lipophilic tend to have a slow elimination.

The amount of time necessary to reduce a certain concentration of a chemical in the plasma by 50% is referred to as the biological half-life. The half-life is determined by plotting a graph of the concentration in the plasma against the time from administration. Although there may be a very rapid rise in plasma concentration following the initial absorption, the curve then takes on a second characteristic of being a straight line regression and the biological half-life is calculated from the straight line part of the curve. An example of the development of a half-life curve of the forest herbicide 2,4,5-T is illustrated in Figure 3 and is taken from the investigations by Gehring (1973). In this experiment, five human volunteers ingested 2,4,5-T at a dosage of 5 mg/kg of body weight and plasma concentrations were then measured at regular intervals following ingestion. In order to develop a straight line curve of excretion, the plasma concentrations are expressed in logarithmic form. In order to determine the half-life of the chemical in human plasma, one can, for example, determine the period of time in which the plasma concentration drops from 40 mcg/ml to 20 mcg/ml. In this case, the half-life of 2,4,5-T is 23.1 hours. This calculation can be expressed in mathematical as well as graphic form. An identical experiment by Sauerhoff (1977) demonstrating the biological half-life of the herbicide 2,4-D is shown in Figure 4. In this

case the biological half-life can be calculated to be
11.6 hours.

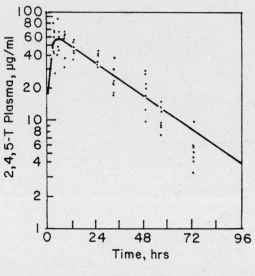

Figure 3

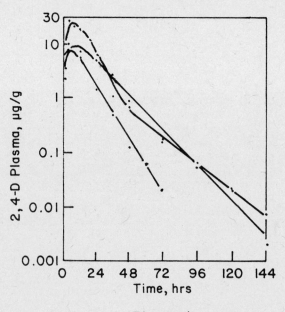

Figure 4

More than just the biological half-life can be calculated from curves such as above. In a review on clinical
pharmacokinetics, Greenblatt and Koch-Wester (1975) discuss this information in more detail. The curve in
Figure 5 is a schematic graph of serum concentrations
versus time and Figure 6 is an actual study performed
showing serum concentrations of the drug chlordiazepoxide
and its active metabolite, desmethylchlordiazepoxide.

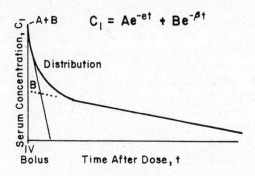

Figure 5

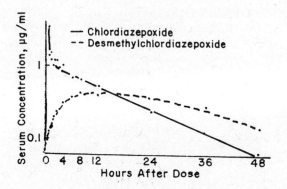

Figure 6

Analysis of these curves can give the following information: distribution half-life, excretion half-life, rate
of body elimination, rate of distribution from vascular
space into tissue, rate of distribution from the tissue
back into the vascular space, volume of distribution
within the body, and rate of metabolism by an organ.

The above types of experiments also demonstrate that
the action of any drug or chemical in the body can, for
purposes of studying its pharmacokinetic behavior, be
divided into compartments. These compartments can vary
greatly in complexity in terms of chemicals getting
from one division to another, but for most purposes,
the body can be divided into a "one-compartment model"
or a "two-compartment model". The one-compartment model
assumes that drugs are instantly and homogeneously distributed within the fluids and tissues of the body and,
therefore, behavior studies can be based entirely upon
dosage and rates of excretion. The more reasonable and
probably realistic model is the two-compartment model
which states that once a chemical is absorbed, distribution occurs to other tissues in the body, sometimes
called the peripheral compartments. Biological action
will occur in the peripheral compartments and excretion
will occur from the peripheral compartment back to the
central compartment of the one-compartment model where
it will then be excreted out of the body. The two-
compartment model explains the change in the downward
slope of the curve shown in Figure 5. If there were
other definitive changes in the slope, it would be an
immediate clue that the drug kinetics was distinctively
more than the two-compartments. Figure 7 demonstrates
the mechanics of the two-compartment model. Point A

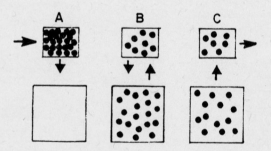

Figure 7

is the instant after rapid ingestion when the drug is held within the central compartment. Point B is the instant when the two compartments come into equilibrium. Point C represents the point when the chemical is returning into the central compartment and then is excreted out of the body.

In addition to studying plasma concentrations versus dosage-time and mechanisms of biological action, another useful parameter is the investigation of the urinary excretion curves following administration of chemicals. Clinically, the establishment of normals of excretion, which are sometimes zero but sometimes are at very low levels, may allow for the diagnosis of either acute or chronic exposure. Follow-up of serial samples gives an indication of the rate of excretion as well as helping to establish any type of recent exposure as levels drop into normal range. Urinary excretion may even be utilized to determine biological half-life, however, for this determination to be accurately made, any chemical under study needs to be excreted almost entirely through the kidneys with no significant excretion occurring via other routes. One of the principal problems in measuring urinary excretion is that the rate of excretion will change depending upon the presence of acute or chronic renal disease. More significantly, excretion of chemicals will change markedly depending upon urinary pH. Thus a small drop in acidity of the urine will lead to considerable retention of drugs, such as in the case of phenoxy herbicides. Conversely, increasing the alkalinity of the urine may lead to increased retention of organic bases. Since the urinary pH may change considerably depending upon diet, these factors will occasionally need to be taken into consideration, particularly in the cases of treatment of excessive chemical exposure when excretion is desired through the kidneys.

An example of measurement of urinary excretion is shown in Figure 8. In this case, the chemical under study was 2,4,5-T (Gehring, 1973). The vertical line on this study now demonstrates the percentage of dose excreted rather than the concentration and is plotted against time. The graph demonstrates nicely some of the distinction between various mammals since, in this case, the biological half-life of rats is calculated to be 13.6 hours as versus dog which is 86.6 hours. Given wide enough safety factors, this type of difference in half-life is usually of little significance in problems of environmental exposure.

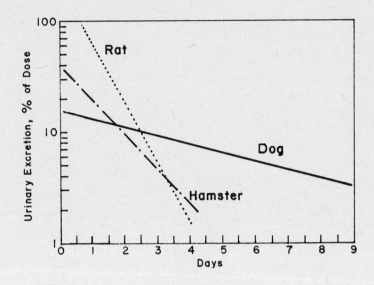

Figure 8

    Although a chemical may remain in the body at the end
of a biological half-life and the dose in then repeated,
the result of consecutive dosages does not lead to for-
ever increasingly higher plasma concentrations. Rather,
the rate of increase gradually decreases until a plateau
is reached, at which time the amount of substance being
ingested will equal the amount of the substance being
excreted. This point is referred to as the equilibrium
concentration and is a useful mechanism in clinical
medicine, as well as in assessing problems of incidental
environmental exposure. As an example, Figure 9, from
Gibaldi and Levy (1976), indicates the drug concentration
in plasma as a function of time during the oral administration of a drug given at 250 mg every six hours with a
biological half-life of nine hours. The C̄ designates
the average steady-state concentration, i.e. the point
at which equilibrium concentration has been reached.
Knowing the pharmacokinetics of any chemical, it is
important to realize that the equilibrium concentration
is accurately predicted without ever having to proceed
through the experiment to make the actual determination
of the equilibrium concentration. In practical terms,
incidental, but chronic, exposure to environmental chemicals may, therefore, lead to a steady-state concentration within the body only if the half-life and dosage

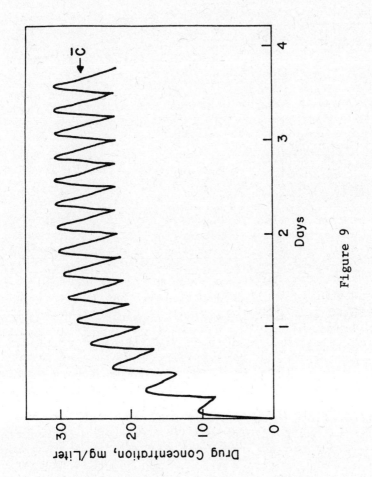

Figure 9

are long enough and high enough respectively. If these
parameters are not exceeded, the chemical will not accrue
to a steady-state concentration.

Although the time required to reach the steady-state
concentration may be relatively long compared to the
biological half-life, it should be remembered that once
exposure to the drug is discontinued, the half-life con-
tinues to operate and that the decline in plasma concentration is directly dependent upon the value of the half-
life and is relatively rapid. Figure 10 demonstrates
such changes. In this case, a drug given intravenously
shows a rise to the equilibrium concentration. Immediately upon discontinuation of the infusion, the drug
concentration will drop very rapidly, dependent upon the
half-life, as shown at the right side of the graph.

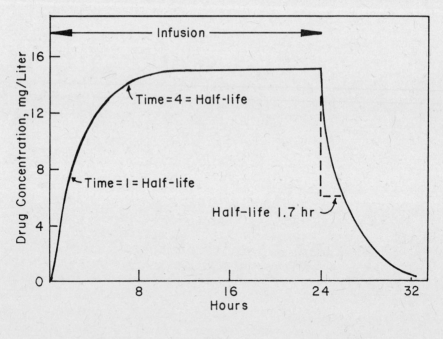

Figure 10

Although the body will excrete all foreign chemicals
or all chemicals which are present in an excessive amount,
again, the nature of the chemical is important. In the
case of those chemicals that are highly lipophilic and,
therefore, generally have a very long half-life, with

repeated exposure, the problem of accumulation may exist. In considering environmental problems, accumulation is particularly serious because of our knowledge that lipophilic chemicals will accumulate in the fat storage areas. Starting with a particular animal of a low form, as one progresses through the food chain, each step upwards in the chain will lead to increasing concentration and storage of the chemical for each particular animal of the food chain. Thus, a chemical which may start out at a very low level in algae may end up at a very high concentration in birds. This was the case which occurred with DDT. In order to avoid such accumulation, one role of the pharmacologist and/or toxicologist is to find chemicals which have essentially the same properties except that they are less lipophilic. In the case of DDT, the chlorine atoms were removed and replaced by methylated hydroxy groups and methoxychlor was thus developed as shown below. This chemical is much more suitable for metabolism and, therefore, is much more easily excreted.

DDT   Methoxychlor

Toxicodynamic Phase

Following individual chemical exposure with subsequent absorption and transportation to a particular tissue in the body, the chemical may then proceed to a toxic effect. However, the mere presence of a chemical at susceptible tissues in not in itself a requirement for the occurrence of a universal toxic effect. Toxic effects occur via well defined biological mechanisms and often the toxic action can be demonstrated. Toxicity to an organism must be the result of some mechanism such as inactivation of enzymes, interference with certain types of protein or small molecule synthesis, interference with oxygen transport or hemoglobin formation, allergic reactions or interference with immune mechanisms, as some common examples. The point is that the clinician has some parameter to measure besides that of history of exposure. Even in the case of a primary injury, such as direct chemical irritation of tissues, these changes can be visualized since the direct irritation usually occurs at the periphery of the body, such as the skin or upper respiratory tract.

Figure 11 (Clayton, 1974) is a graph demonstrating the relationship between the accumulated percent of toxic and nontoxic patients in a study related to total body glycoside (digitalis) concentration. It can be seen that the higher the body concentration, the greater the percentage of patients that express evidence of clinical toxicity. Although this type of information is not always very useful in the examination of a single individual, in the evaluation of numbers of people who have had exposure, these types of studies are very sig- nificant since this type of curve demonstrates that <u>at a low concentration, toxic effects will only be seen in a small percentage of the exposed people.</u> Given a con-

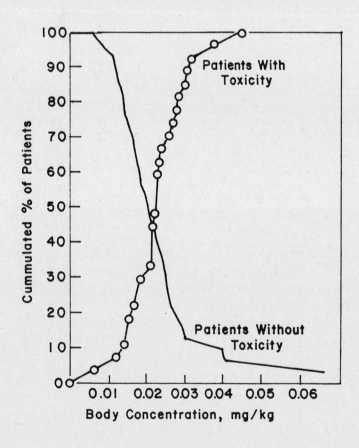

Figure 11

centration which is well below what would be expected to produce a significant percentage of effect, the clinician needs to seek independent answers when faced with a large percentage of people offering complaints from what would appear to be incidental exposure. This concept will be discussed in more detail in the section on Dose-Response.

Dose-Response Relationships

A fundamental principle in the study of chemical action which utilizes classic toxicology methods is the demonstration of what is known as a <u>dose-response</u> relationship. This is a method of graphically illustrating what is known to be the most common and established method of biological response, i.e. the chemical reaction is dependent upon amount in a predictable relationship. By this method, toxicologists allow for the comparison of a chemical action, regardless of type, from one animal to another and hope to allow for distinctions in time. These terms and relationships are discussed below.

<u>Dose</u>: Although dose may be construed to indicate an absolute amount, such as 1 mg or 10 mg, etc., in the field of toxicology, the dosage actually is defined as a ratio rather than an absolute amount. That is, the word dose is an expression of the amount of drug or chemical as related to some other measurement, such as a kg of body weight, surface area, etc. The use of a ratio in expressing dosage allows for direct comparison between animals. Thus, 1 mg/kg given to a rat would be relatively the same dosage as 1 mg/kg given to a monkey or even a larger animal. The use of dosage in this form does imply that the tissue distribution within different animals will be the same regardless of the animal under study and it also assumes that other factors, such as the route of administration, the method of absorption and detoxification, etc., are also similar parameters. Dose-response curves cannot be utilized to compare different families of animals against others. That is, mammals can be compared against mammals, but it is unwise to compare mammals against fish. This is because of the known differences, not only in absorption, but also in metabolism of mammals versus other animals. It should also be noted in defining dosage for toxicology studies that the route of administration must be considered in

comparing and evaluating the experiment. That is, it is important to note whether the route of administration would be subcutaneous, intravenous, intraperitoneal and so forth. Not only is the route of administration important, the amount of the dosage should always be looked at in toxicology studies. Given a large enough dose, any chemical can be harmful and one must always keep in mind the necessity of attempting to relate dose-response experiments to what is, in fact, some sense of proportion to what is occurring in the natural environment.

Response: The response is simply a measurement of some end point in an experimental situation. In this context, this means an easily measured phenomenon in the laboratory, the easiest of which is the death of an animal following a single dosage of the chemical. It is just as realistic, however, although much more difficult experimentally, to measure response by a variety of other parameters, such as a change in some physical measurement, e.g. height or weight; a change in some biochemical parameter, e.g. level of blood sugar, enzyme change, or blood count; or, even some change in social or psychological behavior if the latter can be studied in a quantitative fashion.

The ED_{50}

The ED_{50} is a statistical estimate of the dosage of a chemical that would produce a measured effect on a population of animals 50% of the time. In developing the statistical methods to make this estimate, it is not necessary to use a large population of animals in an experimental study. This is true because of established knowledge of the behavior of biochemical reactions. The experimenter uses test animals which are divided into moderately sized groups of 10-100 animals per unit of dosage given. The dosages are usually given in some geometric or logarithmic manner and experiments are planned in the hope that a small dose will produce either no effect or a minimal effect, whereas a larger dose will produce the same effect in a much greater proportion or percentage of animals.

Given a set of experimental conditions in which groups of animals are given different dosages in an attempt to produce a measureable response, a characteristic type of curve can be plotted on regular graph paper as illustrated

in Figure 12A. In this case, dosage is the horizontal
line and is expressed as mg/kg. The response in the
graph is a measurement of mortality and is expressed as
the vertical line.

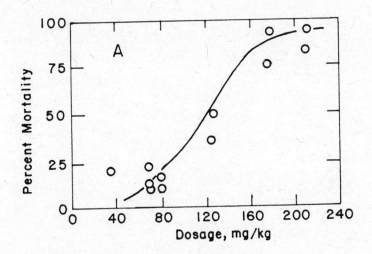

Figure 12A

Even assuming variability of the population, a rather
characteristic S-shaped curve will be developed after
enough experiments. The ED50 can then be read from this
curve and is noted to be that dosage at which 50% of the
animals can be predicted to have responded.

Because the middle part of the curve plotted on arith-
metic paper is frequently non-linear in appearance, this
makes the determination of the 50% level more difficult.
It is, therefore, common to develop the curve further
than shown in Figure 12A by changing it into a logarithmic form such as shown in Figure 12B. In this case, the
S-shaped pattern becomes much more linear in the area
between the 20-80% response and allows for an easier
measurement.

Finally, one can convert both the dosage and response
into logarithmic form and one now has what is referred to
as a log-log curve or a log-normal curve such as shown in
Figure 12C. In this case, the use of the word "log-
normal" does not have the same meaning as "normal" in
usual statistics. In the latter case, one is referring

to "Gaussian" distribution of events, whereas in this case, log-normal sumply refers to an expression of the log-log relationship.

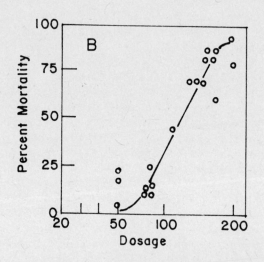

Figure 12B

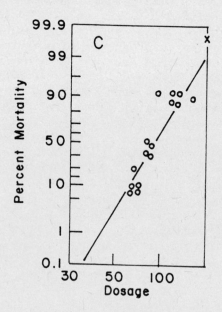

Figure 12C

It is critically important, and one should emphatically note, that the curve in Figure 12C is a straight line and apparently intersects the horizontal line of dosage. In fact, there is a subtlety to this curve which is not always apparent, which is, the zero point for response is never reached. Indeed, it is this lower dosage and lower response area which presents the major difficulty in the study of populations regarding exposure to chemicals, as will be discussed shortly, and it is this part of the curve upon which many environmental issues, as well as the development of regulations, develop from hypothetical rather than factual standpoints. Unfortunately, neither the upper nor the lower portion of the above curves can be studied experimentally because of practical impossibilities in performing the experiments. This will also be explained further in the next section. In summary, what one can understand from the above type of curve is that a percent response, which could be the ED_{10}, the ED_{50} or an ED_{90}, i.e. a dose whereby can be demonstrated that 10%, 50% or 90% respectively of the animals will respond, can be predicted accurately.

It should also be understood that the dosage may be expressed under experimental conditions whereby a chemical may be given either in a single acute dose or in multiple, possibly cumulative or chronic, exposure situations. Furthermore, response can be measured by a variety of different parameters, not only one particular type. The experimenter, as well as the reviewer of scientific literature, must specify, as well as understand, the conditions under which the experiment is being performed. A variety of different investigational methods are utilized. The most common of these is probably the LD_{50} which is the abbreviation meaning 50% lethal dose. In this case, it is defined as 50% of the animals which die at a particular dose and the dosage is usually considered to be a single acute dose. Chronic dosage studies are also performed and require different types of response measurements than death in most experimental situations. In chronic dosage experiments, some attempt is now being made to develop a method of expressing dose-response which also takes into account the interval of time.

The Threshold Concept - and Controversy

Given the accepted fact that biological phenomenon follows a characteristic dosage-response relationship as demonstrated, a great controversy exists over the nature of the curve at that point at which it appears to cross the horizontal line. That is, is there a lowest dosage below which no response can be produced? Utilizing the graph in Figure 13, a number of definitions must first be stated prior to further discussion of this important question.

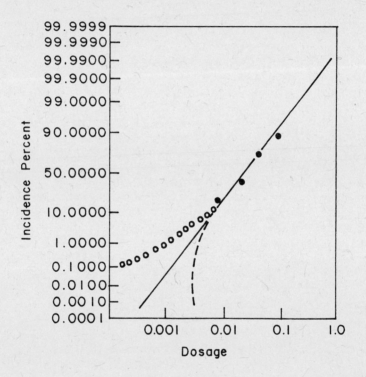

Figure 13

The above curve is an example of data which might be constructed to demonstrate the incidence of tumors in mice following a single dose of some known carcinogen. Both dosage and response are expressed logarithmically. The straight black line which has been constructed represents the true dose-response curve, however, it can be seen that by continually decreasing the dose and lowering

the incidence fraction of response, it would appear that
the curve can never really touch the horizontal line.
(In fact, the curve would have to touch the horizontal
line following the absence of a single molecule of the
chemical.) In practical terms, the incidence fraction
must be stopped at some point and, therefore, if the
straight line dose-response curve were continued, it
would also intersect the horizontal line - or dose - at
a specific point. This point of intersection is referred
to as the threshold. Threshold is thus defined as the
dosage below which no response will occur, i.e. enzyme
response or cancer. In animal experiments, as opposed
to in vitro experiments involving molecules, the above
graph demonstrates that it is impossible for enough
animals to be used in an experiment to statistically
prove the existence of the threshold level. Whereas,
an incidence response of 0.00001 (one in 100,000) would
be impossible to demonstrate in an animal experiment,
the importance of this incidence response is very significant in a large population. That is, in a population
of 200 million, if the incidence response were one in
100,000, this would mean that 2,000 people in a given
period of time would develop a particular disease. Such
issues thus have great meaning in terms of chronic diseases, particularly cancer, birth defects and so forth.
     There are some other characteristics of the dose-
response curve which are frequently referred to. For
example, the lowest dosage at which a response can be
measured is referred to as the least significant effect
level. This term actually has meaning only in the sense
that it is part of the entire dose-response curve and
the restraints of the term are that, particularly with
animal experiments, if more animals were used for each
dose tested, it is conceivable that the least significant
effect level would be lower than that described in the
particular experiment. Directly underneath the least
significant effect level is another term which is frequently used and is the highest dosage given in which no
response is seen. This is referred to as the no observable effect level or the NOEL. Again, this term does
not imply that no further response will occur at low
levels but only that in the particular experimental
situation, this particular dosage with a predetermined
number of animals does not produce an effect. The NOEL
is a commonly used point in toxicology experiments below
which calculations of safety are determined.

Again utilizing the above figure, if the dose-response curve which is developed from experimental data is not a straight line in the lower dosage range and does not transect the dose at some point, what are the alternatives? In fact, the curve can only assume two different directions. In one case, there would be a downward flexure, as expressed by the dashed line. In this case, a threshold would clearly exist and conditions of low dosage would then be of no significance. The alternative is that the curve would bend to the left, as expressed by the dotted line, and this implies that there is a "no threshold" response. Thus, any dose, regardless of size, will produce some type of response in the animal or population of animals and the detection of that response is dependent upon the size of the population and conditions of the experiment.

It is not the intent of this chapter to fully discuss the argument of threshold versus no threshold. It is hoped that the inability to demonstrate a threshold in animal experiments can be perceived from the above discussion. The argument that a threshold exists is also very strong and has been summarized by Kotin (1976), among others. The issue here is not whether the majority of scientists accept or do not accept the threshold hypothesis. The position currently taken in this country, especially with regard to the development of chronic disease and the development of safety factors related to chemical exposures, is that the threshold should be assumed to not exist. Rather, the threshold hypothesis is ignored and instead safety is generally built around a term referred to as the linear-nonthreshold response. The linear-nonthreshold response is the straight line which can be drawn from zero dose and zero incidence response to the last point of observable effect in an experimental dose-response curve, i.e. the least significant effect level. The assessment of safety is then drawn with that type of curve in mind. What constitutes absolute safety is also a highly controversial issue and is discussed in another section. In terms of dose-response curves or in experiments in which a NOEL or a least significant effect level can be defined, an attempt is made to define safety by the use of the dose-response curve. A dose is theorized in which response should occur in only a very small population, such as one response per 100 million subjects. Other factors are, however, clearly important and an attempt is made to take them into account, although this sometimes may be rather subjective. One also considers problems of individual hypersensitivity or allergy (also dose-response related), the amount of production and distribution of the chemicals, variations in host resistance, benefits to society - the so-called cost:benefit ratio - and a variety of other factors. The multiplicity of these factors regarding the question of safety and variety of scientific approaches, besides the use of the dose-response curve, is probably the major reason for the many arguments which seem to occur in this field. Since the lower end of the dose-response curve will never be determined absolutely, it is unlikely that these arguments will cease. Also, it is unfortunate that many chemicals which are currently marketed do not have well defined dose-response curves, at least not in the scientific literature. What occurs is that the least significant effect level or the no observable effect level is utilized as a starting point and safety factors are taken from either of those two points.

Toxicological studies which determine no effect levels or similar parameters are sometimes questioned by the general public since the parameters measured appear to be crude, e.g. weight gain or loss, gross evidence of changes in the furry coat of animals, gross morbidity or gross pathological changes and so forth. Interestingly enough, these studies frequently hold up both in later clinical assessments and when more refined, and therefore more difficult, studies are performed. For example, an interesting comparison of the no effect levels of the organochlorine pesticides when studied from two different parameters has been done by Den Tonkelaar and Van Esch (1974). In this study, a number of organochloride pesticides were given in the diet of rats. The induction of microsomal liver enzymes by different dose levels of these chemicals was studied so that a no effect level was established for each pesticide. This was then compared with the no effect level in the literature, based on the histopathological abnormalities found in the liver from other long-term experiments. Not only was excellent agreement found for the compounds in the study but the no effect level really did not change significantly from the very sensitive study on mixed function oxidases, i.e. stimulation of the smooth endoplasmic reticulum of the liver. Thus the comparison of the no effect level by measuring the weight of the liver, by looking at the optical histopathological changes or by looking at very sensitive systems seen only as as enzyme study or under electron microscopy revealed only small changes in the actual dose-response curve for these compounds.

It is frequently assumed that the younger the age of an animal, the more sensitive that animal will be to pesticide effect. By contrast, studies by Hudson and co-workers (1972) demonstrate that the acute oral toxicity of a pesticide is more related to the type of pesticide studied than to the age of the animal. Extremes of susceptibility can be shown to occur, however the difference in susceptibility is not large in terms of the dose, generally less than three to four fold. In addition, there may be a biphasic type of effect in which the animals have a particular type of response when young and when old but have a different response during the majority of their life. The LD_{50} can, therefore, vary either upwards or downwards depending upon the age of the animal.

Summary

The basic principles of evaluating response of organisms to chemicals by the classical methods of toxicology have been described. It is important to note that biological responses to chemicals can be measured in a predictable and reproducible fashion and that the chemicals produce objective parameters at which to look in a variety of living organisms. Extrapolation to man from these methods usually allows us to make a good assessment of the response in human beings or in our environment. The concept of "threshold" is a critical one and although such thresholds are believed to exist in acute diseases or experimental situations, the ability to demonstrate threshold or no-threshold is presently considered to be an insurmountable problem in the assessment of the relationship of chemicals to such chronic diseases as cancer or birth defects. Despite its limitations, the field of toxicology is objective and follows a scientific method which can be measured and reproduced. It eliminates the purely subjective responses.

References

Clayton, B.D. (1974) Reduction of digitalis glycoside
    intoxication by rational dosing procedures.
    Amer J Hosp Pharm 31:855-865.

Den Tonkelaar, E.M. and G.J. Van Esch (1974) No-effect
    levels of organochlorine pesticides based upon
    induction of microsomal liver enzymes in short-term
    toxicity experiments. Toxicol 2:371-380.

Gehring, P.J. (1973) The fate of 2,4,5-trichlorophenoxy-
    acetic acid (2,4,5-T) following oral administration
    to man. J Toxicol Appl Pharmacol 26:352-361.

Gibaldi, M. and G. Levy (1976) Pharmacokinetics in
    clinical practice. JAMA 235:1987-1992.

Greenblatt, D.J. and J. Koch-Weser (1975) Clinical
    pharmacokinetics. N Eng J Med 293:702-705.

Hudson, R.H., R.K. Tucker and M.A. Haeglel (1972)
    Effect of age on sensitivity: Acute oral toxicity
    of 14 pesticides to mallard ducks of several ages.
    Toxicol Appl Pharmacol 22:556-561.

Kotin, P. (1976) Dose-response relationship and
    threshold concepts. Ann NY Acad Sci 271:22-28.

Sauerhoff, M.W. (1977) The fate of 2,4-dichlorophenoxy-
    acetic acid (2,4-D) following oral administration to
    man. Toxicol 8:3-11.

4

Molecular Biology

Introduction

In this era of an explosion of information coming from new scientific method and the resultant accumulating facts, a recently emerged field, which is producing huge amounts of data, is molecular biology. This discipline helps to explain the basic mechanisms and/or the basic molecular chemistry of the transmission of the life process from one generation to the next as well as trying to explain mechanisms of change within living organisms during the life span of the organism. Molecular biology is such a new field, and changes are occurring within the field so rapidly, that scientists in other disciplines often find themselves relatively poorly trained in this field or unable to stay abreast of the advances. The molecular biologists criticize their scientific peers for this and, conversely, molecular biologists are criticized for have too narrow a perspective and of over-emphasizing the importance of their discipline. Intriguingly, molecular biologists consider the gene, i.e. the fundamental life-unit that controls our heritage, man's most important possession. This is philosophically intriguing because most people consider life itself, the process of present living, more important than the process for controlling future generations of life. The use of agricultural chemicals can be looked at from both viewpoints: chemicals clearly affect the present day quality of life in that they allow much greater agricultural production by their use and therefore improve the current quality of life; some chemicals also have the potential to affect the future quality of life by interfering with the world's genetic make-up and potentially producing irreversible, detrimental changes.

Chemical expressions of future change use terms such as mutagens, teratogens, and carcinogens, among others. These terms now require definition before proceeding.

Definitions

Mutagen
: Physical or chemical agents, such as radiation, heat, or alkylating or deaminating agents, which raise the frequency of mutation greatly above the spontaneous background level.

Carcinogen
: An agent that induces cancer.

Teratogen
: An agent that induces birth defects.

Chromosomes
: Threadlike structures into which the hereditary material of cells and viruses is associated.

Genome
: Single set of chromosomes, with their associated genes.

DNA
: The genetic material of all cells.

The remainder of this chapter will discuss the measurement of molecular biological changes in tissue, i.e. measurement of a mutagen or a carcinogen and so forth. The methodology is still in a developing stage with new tests being developed regularly. This chapter will also discuss the methods and the difficulties of assessing genetic changes which might be occurring in the human population. Most of these latter fall into the field of clinical epidemiology and are subject to difficulties related to collection of data and statistical analysis.

Mutagenesis

It is well established that if man is to continue to enjoy a complex society, along with the benefits there will also be certain hazards which we introduce as a secondary and usually undesirable effect. It is clear that a wide variety of chemicals occur in the environment both naturally and as a result of man-made pollution and that some of these chemicals are mutagens. Since these mutagens have the potential of producing changes in our genetic make-up which may not be manifested for several generations, the importance of this particular issue is paramount. Although medicine has made remarkable progress in the field of acute disease care, such as infectious disease, the problems of the chronic diseases are not only with us but relatively are increasing as a cause of human disability. Similarly, the role of genetic illness is now becoming much more apparent with a minimum percentage of all illness which has a genetic factor being somewhere in the range of six percent. Since mutation consists of the abrupt heritable change which occurs in the composition arrangement of genes (DNA), how important are these changes to the human race? It is clear that some mutations may produce effects of little or no consequence and that certain types of mutations are even advantageous to mankind. On the other hand, most mutations which produce effects which are large enough to be measurable are considered deleterious.

An important problem is to determine how one measures mutational changes which are occurring. This can be done through genetic screening and genetic clinics which do, in fact, measure the incidence of certain genetically determined diseases as they occur in the newborn or may even occur in the adult population. The Public Health Service and state Departments of Health all have Departments of Vital Statistics which give us some idea of the incidence of a variety of diseases. For example, we do know the number of birth defects which occur in a state per annum, the number of neonatal mortalities, the incidence of neonatal morbidity, the rate of fetal death and so forth. Such statistics are available and can be used to answer certain types of questions which we ask.

In general, any artifically increased mutation rate is more likely to produce a general decline in the genetic health of our population rather than an improvement. Since we are usually unable to cure a genetic disease, it is desirable to keep the rate of mutations occurring in our society at as low a level as possible and not significantly raise the naturally occurring spontaneous rate of mutation. Thus, one way of protecting against mutagenic chemicals is simply to avoid them as much as possible. To do so does not simply mean that all mutagenic chemicals must be arbitrarily eliminated from the envi-

ronment. We now get into problems of the most basic
scientific nature, e.g. what is the mechanism of mutation, what are reliable screening methods in the population, what is the nature of the dose-response, what is
the reliability of pre-tested methods and so on.

Screening Systems - Ideal

If we rely upon screening systems of the human population to determine mutagenic changes occurring, it is
apparent that by the time such effects are measurable,
the mutagenic chemical will already have been introduced
into our environment. It is, therefore, highly important
that some system be developed which identifies environmental mutagens as a specific cause of certain types of
abnormalities and furthermore, that this identification
can be performed accurately and rapidly in systems prior
to that time when the chemical is being introduced into
society. The characteristics of the ideal screening
system have been described.
First of all, the system should have both sensitivity
and reproducibility. By sensitivity, we mean that the
system should be able to detect a very small mutational
effect, i.e. one that would produce even a small increase
over the spontaneous human mutation rate. This means
that the system must contain a large number of organisms
or animals in order to have statistical accuracy. Reproducibility must occur in any scientific method since this
is the only way that one can demonstrate that a result is
valid and not simply chance. (As an aside, one common
problem occurs when the public is informed of the results
of a single laboratory test which may appear to be either
favorable or unfavorable toward a chemical. These results are taken as fact prior to the opportunity for any
other scientist to reproduce the experiment in order to
test its validity.) Next, the ideal screening system
should be able to detect the whole mutagenic spectrum.
While this at first seems like a task of impossible magnitude, the fact that the genes do act in concordance
with basic chemistry and that the genetic material (DNA)
has been fairly well established, allows us to make, at
least in principle, some statement about the mutagenicity
of a compound as effected in any organism. Thus when a
DNA change may occur in a bacteria, while we cannot apply
this change directly to some genetic change which may
occur in a human being, the fact that the change occurred

at all does have a significance even though the absolute
importance or extrapolation to man cannot be stated with
assurance. Studies on man would indicate an average
mutation rate of 10^{-5} to 10^{-6} per locus per sexual generation. Since comparisons made between the DNA of small
organisms, such as Drosophila fruit fly, versus man indicate that the DNA in man has approximately 10^{5} loci for
the genome, it appears as though one mutation per genome
per human sexual generation occurs (by comparing against
the known spontaneous mutation rate of the Drosophila).
By comparing the fruit fly system to man, one can develop
basic units for application to man. The first is the
rate-doubling concentration, i.e. that concentration of a
chemical that produces twice the genetic damage as occurs
spontaneously in the same period of time in a particular
test system. The second is the rem equivalent chemical
(REC), i.e. that dose or product of concentration multi-
plied by time which produces an amount of genetic damage
equal to that produced by one rem (radiation-equivalent-
man) of chronic irradiation. While it is difficult to
extrapolate from this test system directly to man, it is
believed, at this time, that the effects of radiation are
remarkably constant in diverse biological systems and
that this system can be used on lower test animals.

Metabolic factors influencing mutagens must be considered since many chemicals may be inert as they are distributed in the environment but may be changed as they
are metabolized in the body or, conversely, many chemicals
may be active initially and then metabolize in an inert
product. Thus any examination in terms of potential
mutagenicity of a particular chemical has to include an
analysis of its metabolic fate as well as simply study of
the chemical on some particular system.

Dosimetry must also be considered in mutagen studies.
The amount of chemical being introduced, the route of
absorption, and the concentration actually reached at the
target tissues are all factors in the dose assessment.
Studies on routes of absorption should be as realistic
and natural as possible since it is unlikely that man will
be dosed by some route in which a needle is injected into
the abdominal cavity and the drug injected thereto. If
the chemical has an effect upon a particular organ, such
as the gonads, the concentration actually achieved by the
chemical at that particular organ is of more importance
than the actual amount to which the test organism has been
subjected. Quantitative extrapolation of these types of
test systems must not be based simply upon any type of

single dose test but must, instead, be based upon dose-
response curves as occurs in the basic science of toxicology. At the moment, it should be assumed that there
is no such thing as a threshold level to a mutagen in
any system and that the best practice, when extrapolating
from dose-response curves, is to assume a linear no
threshold response from the no observable effect level to
the zero dosage level. If safety factors are then taken
into account with this type of developed dose-response
curve, the risk to society would at least not be under-
estimated.

Finally, the ideal screening system should be able to
test mutagen interactions, i.e. the likelihood of two
mutagens reacting either synergistically or antagonistically with each other. We do not know this type of
information nor, indeed, could we really develop it since
there are so many mutagens and the possibilities of testing all mutagens against each other for some type of interaction is practically impossible. It is assumed,
until information to the contrary may sometime develop,
that all mutagens produce simple additive effects at the
lower exposure levels. This seems to be a reasonable,
albeit conservative, assumption.

In order to detect as much of the mutagenic spectrum
as possible, certain types of mutations that are predicted to occur are monitored in the following manner: 1)
changes in chromosome number, 2) changes resulting from
chromosome breaks, 3) single gene mutations, i.e. point
mutations, and 4) studies on the basic units and the
spontaneous baseline rate of mutation change.

Currently Employed Screening Systems

While the above describes the ideal type of screening
systems, the actual types of systems which we have do not
meet all of the above desired characteristics. Examples
of presently used systems are described in the following
table.

Screening System

Category	Organism
Bacterial	Salmonella typhimurium
	Escherichia coli
Fungal	Neurospora crassa
	Asperigillus nidulans
	Yeasts
Plant	Vicia faba
	Tradescantia paludosa
Insect	Drosophila melanogaster
	Habrobracon juglandis
	Bombyx mori
Mammalian cell culture	Chinese hamster
	Mouse lymphoma
Intact mammal	Mouse
	Rat
	Man

It must be emphasized that a mutational change in any one system does not necessarily mean that a mutational change will also occur in man. However, as a group, the systems can all be used. The more likely that a chemical will involve a number of systems, the more likely that it will also be detrimental to man. Furthermore, certain systems, such as the test for mutagenicity in bacteria, can be shown to have a certain statistical correlation against predictable effects in human beings although, again, the detection of a mutagen in one system always requires the validity by further experimentation in other systems. Preferably, these studies are on whole animals, since the whole animal is still considered one of the more valuable methods of studying genetic changes. The operational characteristics of these systems quickly show that a bacterial system may only take a matter of several days in order to detect a genetic change, whereas, studies on mammals may require a number of months or years. Finally, the identification of a compound as a mutagen is only the first step in estimating the hazard it may pose to man and a variety of additional information is re-

quired, such as the amount and distribution of the chemical in the environment, its persistence, exposure of the
human being, metabolic disposition and the effect of
other environmental factors in the chemical per se.

Studies by Ercegovich and Rashid (1977) upon the mutagenic effect of 70 pesticides as evaluated in five strains
of Salmonella typhimurium, alone, with and without activation by liver microsomal enzymes are illustrated below.

Non-Mutagenic	Weak Mutagens	Mutagenic	Weak Mutagens (only after activation)
Chlordane	Benomyl	Captan	Aldicarb
2,4-D	Dieldrin	Dimethoate	Bromopropylate
Endrin	Lindane		Chlordimeform
Fenazaflor	Thiabeneazole		Furidazole
Guthion			Heptachlor
Terrazole			Carbaryl
Zolone			Methyl Parathion

Chemicals tested only without activation gave the following results:

Non-Mutagens	Weak Mutagens	Strong Mutagens
Amitrole	Ametryne	DDT
Atratone	2,4-D Butyl Ester	4-Chloro-o-toluidine
Atrizine	Desmedipham	2,4-D Ethyl Ester
Propham	Maleic Hydrazide	1-Naphthol Isothymol
Simazine	Picloram	
Simatone	Promacarb	
Simetryne		
2,4,5-T		
Beta-Carbaryl		

Risk Analysis

The above describes the fundamental methods of mutagen
screening in test systems in order to detect those chemicals which might be potential mutagens and, therefore,
harmful to man. Trying to apply such mutagen systems to
man, leads to two major problems: the choice of methods
for quantitatively extrapolating from test systems to
man, and, the choice of criteria for deciding what are

the acceptable versus the unacceptable risks.

When one attempts to extrapolate test systems to their significance in man, as a general principle it has been considered most desirable to extrapolate to man from those systems which are closest to man - such as mammalian tests. While there is a good correlation between tests in microbial systems, at this time these tests are used mainly as indicators for further experiments. Presently, there is no reliable method of doing a quantitative extrapolation from any test system to man and the best that can be done is to use either the factor of increase over the spontaneous background or the ratio of chemical to radiation mutagenesis.

We are, therefore, again left with the question of asking how much and how many chemical mutations are safe, i.e. acceptable risk to society (see Part I, Chapter 3). One principle that is clear in this regard is that no risk whatsoever is the acceptable response when the mutagenic compound presents no clear benefits, or, when an alternative non-mutagenic compound or method is available at no significantly increased social or economic cost. Furtherfore, when a useful compound that is already in distribution is discovered to be mutagenic, efforts should be made to replace it with a less hazardous compound which already exists or to attempt to develop some type of substitute.

We are frequently faced with the problem of developing some type of risk:benefit ratio. This is difficult to do in any quantitative way although every attempt should be made to do so.

The current recommendations of the Environmental Mutagen Society of the United States are that a maximum limit of a 12.5% increase over the present spontaneous mutational load should be the most upward allowable adjustment. This is an important recommendation which should be followed but one should also recognize the difficulties in determining not only the present spontaneous mutation load but also the difficulties in knowing what chemicals exist in our environment which may be mutagens. The Environmental Mutagen Society further goes on to recommend that no single mutagenic agent should be allowed to exceed 10% of the five REC budget alloted to all mutagenic agents and that this limit should be absolute with no compound producing even substantial benefits to be disseminated beyond a level producing this effect.

The above recommendations are directed at the average population. Recognizing that certain industrial and

agricultural workers may be more heavily exposed, the
Environmental Mutagen Society then proceeds to recommend
that the maximum permissible mutagenic exposure to individuals who are still within their reproductive life span
be limited to a ten-fold excess over the average maximum
permissible exposure level. They are careful to emphasize that this level of exposure might more than double
the workers genetic risk expectancy and that, therefore,
these workers should be informed of their increased risk
status. Furthermore, it is strictly understood that
these individuals should be averaged in with the entire
population so that there is still not an increase above
the recommended limit of 12.5%.

The importance of determining mutagenic chemicals and
of assessing risk has not gone unnoticed on the international level. This important issue has led the International Association of Environmental Mutagen Societies
to establish an International Commission For Protection
Against Environmental Mutagens and Carcinogens (ICPEMC).
The ICPEMC was organized in January of 1977 and six tasks
which were felt to be of compelling importance were
identified:

1. The development, validation, application
    and comparison of short-term screening
    systems for the identification and char-
    acterization of chemical mutagens and
    carcinogens.

2. The relation between carcinogenesis
    and mutagenesis.

3. The establishment of a registry of national
    regulatory principles and actions.

4. The formulation of general principles
    for developing risk estimates that may
    serve as a basis for setting maximum
    exposure limits.

5. A survey of epidemiology studies on those
    sections of the human population that
    are being exposed to mutagenic and car-
    cinogenic agents.

6. A continuing review of the state of our
    knowledge with regard to levels of chronic
    and acute exposure to specific chemical.

Monitoring For Genetic Effects in Man

Why are we concerned with the introduction of mutagenic (and carcinogenic) chemicals into our environment?
And, if there is a cause for concern, how can we effectively monitor any deleterious effects before they become
significant, or, can we determine if there is such a
thing as a "safe level"?
We are concerned about the possibility of increased
mutation rates for two reasons. First, it is the intui-
tive belief of many geneticists that the mutation rate of
a species, as presently established through the operation
of the process of natural selection, should be close to
the optimum for that species. It is possible that any
changes in the process of natural selection may be harmful. Second, experimental demonstrations, particularly
in the fruit fly Drosophila, have shown that most induced
mutations do, indeed, have deleterious effects. Thus,
there is a significant feeling for a cautious approach
and, certainly, an obvious need to continually evaluate
the situation.
In practice, the present techniques for laboratory
screening of mutagenicity in chemicals follows a multiple
tier test system. The first level involves tests with
bacteria, such as the Ames test. The second level of the
tier involves the use of special strains of the Drosophila
fruit fly. Finally, the third level generally involves
cultured mammalian cells. At each level, a decision is
made as to whether there are indications to proceed further. If the final screen results are still not conclusive, further studies can be made in whole mammalian test
systems. The latter is by far the most difficult in terms
of time and expense to perform although whole mammal test
systems may independently be used to assess the possibility of mutagenic effects and completely bypass the initial
screening procedures. The efficacy of all of the above
systems is made more complex because any single chemical
which is tested may be converted by man's metabolism into
more or to less dangerous chemicals and also by the fact
that the chemicals may act either synergistically or
antagonistically.
We have, therefore, evolved three principal approaches
which are used to detect an increasing germinal mutational rate in human populations - as opposed to laboratory
experiments.

"Population Characteristics" Approach

The "population characteristics" approach uses
changes in such demographic events as frequency of still-
births, mean birth weight, frequency of congenital defect, sex ratio, death rates during the early years of
life, and physical growth and development during infancy
and childhood as indications of an increase (or decrease)
in mutation rates. The argument that changes in mutation
rates should be reflected in these indicators is sound.
The problem is that the relationship between any change
in the indicator and the underlying change in mutation
rate cannot always be clearly made. Furthermore, any
indicator will necessarily be influenced by many other
exogenous factors in the environment which operate on
both the mother and the child. A suitable control group
must also be available and establishing such control
groups is difficult since one must match as many parameters in an "exposed" group as there are in the "control"
group, i.e. age, sex, occupation, etc.

"Sentinel Phenotypes" Approach

The "sentinel phenotype" approach monitors a defined
population (or contrast to suitable population) for
changes in the rate of occurrence of isolated cases
(within the family) of certain phenotypes likely to have
resulted from a dominant mutation in a germ cell. That
is, certain typical genetic diseases such as hemophilia,
neurofibromatosis, congenital polycystic disease of the
kidneys, etc. are used as markers of mutation rates.
The use of this approach is difficult since the rates
which presently exist in the population are not always
known and are sometimes very difficult to determine,
particularly in the cases of very rare diseases. Certain
cases of change in sentinel phenotypes could simply
represent non-genetic developmental accidents, could be
the result of somatic mutation as opposed to germ cell
mutation, or could represent some type of recessive
inheritance. Furthermore, mutation at any one of several
different genetic loci could result in clinically indis-
tinguishable phenotypes, i.e. a change in a single locus
might result in more than one type of disease expression
and thereby further dilute the problem of collecting
statistics. On the practical side, a major problem in
selecting any sentinel phenotype is to develop clear-cut

diagnostic criteria by which the disease is definitely
established in the young person and also to establish a
large scale registration system which could be available.
Finally, critical in the study of sentinel phenotypes is
the problem of the population size which must be kept
under intensive surveillance in order to detect defects
of at least a 50% increase in mutation rates. In other
words, if an increase in 50 appearances per 100,000
births to 75 per 100,000 has, in fact, occurred, the
question is how many births must be monitored to be confident of detecting an increase at a desired statistical
level? A crude birth rate of 20 per 100,000 population
requires a study population of between six and nine
million simply to detect an effect on a year to year
basis.

Biochemical Approach

Recent advances in our ability to isolate and charac-
terize a wide variety of human proteins, coupled with the
knowledge of the genetic code and its relationship to
amino acid sequences, seem to permit us to circumvent
some of the difficulties involved in studying whole populations (sometimes referred to as "point" mutations or
changes in the gross organismic phenotype). It is now
possible and, indeed, a frequent practice to examine
human tissue specimens of placental cord blood, blood, or
urine specimens from children in order to detect the
variation in serum or blood proteins. When a variant is
encountered, it may be possible to determine by suitable
family studies whether the variation was inherited from
one parent or the other, or whether both parents were
normal and the variant thus resulted from a mutation.
The technology of this field is still evolving, although
rapidly. Examples of such diseases are alpha 1-antitrip-
sin deficiencies, pseudocholinesterase deficiencies,
glucose-6-phosphate dehydrogenase deficiency and so on.
At the present time, genetic clinics in this country are
capable of following and treating such types of people
but statistics on incidence, and particularly incidence
changes, are not established. Setting up biochemical
monitoring which could be based either upon the contrast
of the progeny of "high risk" parents versus the progeny
of "control" groups, or on a continuous monitoring system
in which time trends are studied in a "typical" population
will be difficult. A huge number of observations will be

required. For example, if we wish to detect a 50%
increase in the frequency of mutations at a 0.05 or 0.01
significance level, i.e. an increase of an estimated
20 mutations per 100,000 births to 30 per 100,000 births,
then the following populations will need to be studied.
At the 0.05 significance level, two samples, each containing 313,000 persons, or, at the 0.01 significance
level, 508,000 persons per sample would be required.
Even with automation, it is estimated that a 313,000
person determination would represent the annual output
of at least 200 technicians and 25 supervisory scientists
at a minimum. Recalling that if the crude birth rate is
about 20 per 100,000, then the actual sample which would
be required would be in the range of 15 to 25 million
persons (parents).

In addition to the complexities of setting up such
type of monitoring programs as described above, it should
be apparent that the cost of such programs will be substantial. In addition, the interpretation of data is
also considered to be rather dangerous because a statistically significant finding which is interpreted as
"negative" can result in false reassurance. This would
be particularly true in the case of sample sizes which
are small. Perhaps most important in assessing such
studies is the continued recognition that any increase
or decrease in mutation rates which may be found must
still be clearly identified with the responsible agent or
agents from among the many possible mutagens and other
factors. An interface must exist between studies of
human populations and laboratory experimentation. Most
people feel laboratory studies are probably best extrapolated to humans by studying those particular groups who
have an unusually high exposure to a potential mutagen,
such as occupationally exposed workers.

Carcinogenesis

Molecular Biologists' Viewpoint of Carcinogenesis

The concept that cancer would arise from mutations in
somatic (as opposed to sex-linked) cells was postulated
long before knowledge of the molecular structure of the
genetic material, DNA, was known. The idea was introduced to account for two features of cancerous growth in
man: 1) the unlimited variety of tumor types, and, 2)
the fact that upon cell division, daughter cells maintain

their neoplastic properties. For some time, it was
thought impossible to prove or disprove the somatic
mutation theory since classical Mendelian analysis could
not be applied to somatic cells. Thus, indirect methods
for testing the theory of somatic mutation as a cause of
carcinogenesis were attempted. One approach was to
analyze cancer incidence curves with respect to age in an
attempt to determine whether a mathematical formula would
fit the data - thus assuming a sequence of random mutations. The second indirect approach was to seek a correlation between the mutagenic and carcinogenic action
among chemical compounds that were already known to have
one or the other property.

In the case of experimental carcinogenesis in mice,
it was found that two consecutive random mutations were
needed, or five to six non-consecutive, non-random mutations were needed for cancer development. In human beings, retinoblastoma was shown to be caused by two
mutational events. In the dominantly inherited form,
one mutation was inherited via germinal cells and the
second mutation occurred in somatic cells. In the non-
hereditary form, both mutations occurred in the somatic
cells. The above data suggested, but did not prove,
that the theory for multiple random mutation for cancer
development appeared correct. The practical application
of this theory is that carcinogenesis does not occur
after a single "hit" upon DNA but suggests that multiple
exposures must occur leading to more than one mutation.

Attempts were made to correlate the mutagenic versus
carcinogenic activity of chemical compounds. Early, a
correlation could not be found but it is now believed
that many, and perhaps all, chemical carcinogens are
potential mutagens. Many, but probably not all, mutagens
are potential carcinogens. Of critical importance is the
electrophilic nature of these chemicals - in order for
them to react with DNA as well as cell constituents other
than DNA.

Molecular Basis For Carcinogenesis

Every biological trait of a cell, i.e. normal versus
abnormal or cancerous, must be the result of some interaction of both a genetic nature and environmental factors.
The future development of a cell will depend upon both of
these predispositions. Thus, "normal" DNA may also have
environmentally induced effect to become abnormal. The

genetic influenced disease may be an expression of the
individual to expected and unavoidable environmental
factors, such as the predisposition to handle drug-
metabolism differently than "normal" individuals. It is
believed important to recognize that when any potentially
carcinogenic molecular change occurs in the DNA molecule,
the change could be permanent or temporary. In the latter
case, the possibility of DNA repair must be taken into
account as part of the mechanism which protects the biological unit.

It is thus apparent that carcinogenesis is a complex
process involving both the host and the environment.
Furthermore, it is believed to involve at least a two-
stage process to reach the clinical stage. The first of
these is the initiation of a normal cell to a pre-cancerous cell and the second, is the promotion of proliferation
of the pre-cancerous cells to a clinical stage. Both
stages are, in fact, needed and it is not simply enough
to change a DNA molecule into a pre-malignant cell by some
chemical interaction for a clinical disease to develop.
It is believed that if the DNA molecule has been subjected to initiation leading to a pre-cancerous cell, then if
the promotion mechanism does not occur, the altered DNA
molecule will act as a substrate for various types of DNA
repair. The tumor promoter appears to be a chemical
agent or physical condition which alters the repair mechanism. In summary, the ultimate appearance of a tumor is
probably the end result of many genetic regulatory mechanisms involving molecular, biochemical and cellular
systems, in which the ability for DNA to repair itself
may have been severely impaired. Repairing systems do
exist and what needs to be determined is exactly how much
of a role a DNA repair system plays in the process leading to mutagenesis or carcinogenesis.

Viewed within the summary of the above complex frame-
work, Trosko and Chu (1975) suggest that

> "the goal of a total prevention of cancer
> and the development of a universal therapy
> for the cure of cancer will be extremely
> difficult, if not impossible, to obtain
> .....there are many steps at which genetic
> variability could lead to the genetic
> predisposition to cancer, as well as many
> levels by which certain environmental
> factors can enhance the carcinogenic and
> aging processes."

Dose-Response Controversy and Cancer

Although the construction of dose-response curves is
readily understandable and not argumentative, the presence of a threshold or what happens to the curve below
the observable effect in a laboratory experiment is a
subject of heated debate. Indeed, if this issue could
be solved, much, if not all, of the controversy involving
the use of toxic chemicals would quickly disappear. The
arguments concerning dose-response curves and the existence of thresholds has been summarized by Maugh (1978)
with a quick rejoinder by Hooper, Harris and Ames (1979).
In particular, the question of what happens to an individual after exposure to a very low dose of a carcinogen, or
to another difficult factor to measure, such as a teratogenic chemical, is the prime issue in the question of safe
uses of agricultural chemicals. The difficulty of determining whether or not thresholds exist or whether or not
the curve bends gradually to the left cannot be satisfied
readily from animal experimentation. The principal reason
behind this statement is the necessity to use numbers of
animals in experiments which are well beyond what is
practical. The problem is then further confounded by the
need to extrapolate directly from limited animal experiments to health effects from human exposure. This type
of extrapolation is an assumption and its value in a pre-
dictive sense has been questioned. A major issue is the
yet unanswered question of the mechanism of carcinogenesis. Those scientists opposed to the concept of a
threshold argue for the single-event or "one-hit"
hypothesis which assumes that cancer or some other
genetic change results from the interaction of one
molecule of a carcinogen with one molecule of DNA at
some critical point. In this case, the dose-response
curve would start at zero and continue in a more or less
straight line as the dosage increased. Proponents of the
threshold model believe that there are a variety of
events which occur prior to the actual induction, or at
least the expression, of a tumor or other illness and
therefore, low dosage exposure is not an event of significance. Unfortunately, at the dosages at which this
phenomenon needs to be studied, the number of animals
needed to satisfy the scientific experiment is impossible
to utilize. Therefore, all dose-response curves based
upon animal experiments tend to look the same - and thereby skirt the question. In human beings, the question can
only be answered by long-term epidemiological studies

upon exposed populations, and also require carefully
selected control populations. These studies will
obviously take a number of years and, if the suspected
agent were truly an offender, the continued use of the
chemical might simply lead to a type of "head count" of
death or illness. Therefore, threshold opponents believe
it is reasonable to take appropriate legislative action
to ban chemicals or restrict their use based upon the
preliminary and non-conclusive information derived from
experimental animal systems. In this case, "safety" is
"predicted" by the use of an animal test system in which
animals are fed chemicals at high exposure levels and
observed for the development of a carcinogenic event. If
one assumes that a threshold does not exist, the extrapolation of this kind of data to man can be expressed as
follows. If an animal test system contains 100 rats that
are fed a chemical at a dosage of 1% of the diet, and if
none of these animals develop a cancer, we can then only
be 99% confident that the chemical is not a carcinogen in
a large population at an incidence of $4\frac{1}{2}\%$ or less.
Extrapolating directly to humans, if an exposure level
would then be allowed of only 10 parts per million in the
human diet - as opposed to the 1% in the rats - the
exposure risk to humans would be 5×10^{-5}. While this
appears to be rather small, if one recognizes that the
population of the United States is at least 200 million,
this would yield a population of 10,000 that would be
developing cancer as the result of the chemical exposure.
To state this in a different way, a negative test result
with 100 animals fed a carcinogenic chemical at a concentration of 1% in the diet tells us only that a human
population of less than 10,000 people might contract
cancer if everyone in this country were exposed to the
chemical at the concentration of 10 parts per million -
assuming similar reactions in experimental animals and
humans.

Supporters of the threshold concept point to a variety
of existing long-term studies in occupationally exposed
workers which are already in existence and which do not
show increased evidence of cancer on exposed populations.
In addition, present concepts of carcinogenesis indicate
to most people that a variety of events, rather than a
single event of "one-hit", is a more plausible explanation of the mechanism of carcinogenesis. Also, the
threshold hypothesis may be supported by the relationship
between the dose of a carcinogen and the latent period
between exposure and the initiation of tumor growth.

Generally, it is believed that the latent period increases as the dose is reduced. That is, at a very low dose, the latent period would be longer than any individual would live and, therefore, the cancer would not develop. In effect, this represents a type of practical threshold based upon the inability of the human to live long enough to develop cancer from the offending agent.

It would seem that in the future, regulatory agencies will have to determine whether or not to litigate all carcinogens out of our society - and we seem to be living with an ever increasingly large number of them - or to assume that there is a relatively hazard-free dosage at which humans can be exposed to harmful agents. This assessment will be based largely upon existing dose-response curves and the development of safety guidelines for maximum allowable exposure.

A discussion of the low-dose extrapolation problem, i.e. estimating safe dose levels of chemicals which are believed to be carcinogenic, can be found in detail in other papers, notably by Wahrendorf (1979) or by Van Ryzin (1980). The variety of models, i.e. single hit, multiple hit, multiple stage, etc. approaches to looking at the problem, are discussed with the mathematical formulae and the significance of different approaches referrable to human health predictions.

Role of Regulatory Agencies

Eventually, a regulatory agency must take a position regarding the "safety" of any chemical. This may be done with definitive, or only preliminary, data of a scientific nature. At the present time, most agencies prefer to take a very cautious stand and to err on the side of heavy protection for humans. The following quote from the position of the National Cancer Institute as expressed in "Human Health Considerations of Carcinogenic Organic Chemicals Contaminants in Drinking Water" is an example of present thinking.

> "The National Cancer Institute, working
> collaboratively with the Environmental
> Protection Agency, compiled - from USA
> and European reports - a list of over 1700
> organic compounds found in water. These
> compounds have been found in various kinds
> of water ranging from raw water and indus-

trial effluents to drinking water at the
tap. The question with respect to these
compounds is what do they do?

"Although there is some duplication
in listing of carcinogens and mutagens,
there are currently 23 carcinogens or
suspected carcinogens, 30 mutagens or
suspected mutagens, and 11 promoters in
drinking water identified from a 1976
list of organic compounds found in drinking water in the United States.

"Many of the organic contaminants
identified in drinking water such as
chloroform, carbon tetrachloride, tri-
chloroethylene, 1,2-dibromoethane, vinyl
chloride, bis(2-chlorethyl) ether and
others, have been proven as carcinogens
in bioassays with the rodent (rat and
mouse) in several laboratories, including
the National Cancer Institute. Additional
evidence is provided from studies on marine
animals which showed a four-fold tumor
incidence in fish from polluted waters
compared to those from less polluted waters.

"Two sets of studies have been done
looking for a relationship in humans
between trihalomethanes and possible
increases in cancer. The first set used
presumed measures of chlorination, i.e.
surface (likely to be chlorinated, therefore likely to contain trihalomethanes)
water vs. ground water (unlikely to be
chlorinated). The second set used actual
measures of the levels of trihalomethanes
- the EPA's National Organics Reconnaissance
Survey studies, and the EPA Region V studies.

"Nine of ten studies which involved the
indirect indicators showed a number of
statistically significant associations
between water quality and cancer. The
10th study (Los Angeles) failed to identify any positive associations; however,
it appeared to have limitations greater
than those of any of the other studies,
most particularly problems of great
population movement.

"The three 'quantitative' studies
(with measures of trihalomethane level)

lead to the tentative conclusion that bladder cancer, and perhaps large intestine cancers, are correlated with trihalomethane in the water. The sites found positive in these studies are different from the sites (liver and kidney) found in the animal studies. One of the quantitative studies leads to the conclusion that an increase of 100 ug/l of chloroform in water could lead to an increase in cancer rates as follows:

	Men	Women
Bladder	1.3 to 7.5%	5.3 to 10%
Large Intestine	4.0 to 8.5%	3.0 to 7.5%

"None of the authors of any of these studies asserts that the trihalomethane-cancer association is proved. But on a weight-of-evidence basis one should have a high index of suspicion.
"In the interest of cancer prevention, it seems to be prudent to control and/or reduce the exposures to drinking water carcinogenic contaminants. The proposed regulation to set a maximum contaminant level of 100 parts per billion for total trihalomethanes is a constructive public health measure in that direction. Measures taken to control large classes of contaminants are likely to be useful in reducing levels of material whose carcinogenic or mutagenic potential is still unknown."

The NCI position paper drew the following conclusions and recommendations.

1. Animal experimental data has demonstrated that many of the organic contaminants in water are carcinogens.

2. Evidence of carcinogenicity of a similar material in animals has, in several instances, been followed by similar evidence in humans. Conversely, all but one or two human carcinogens have been shown to produce cancer in animals.

3. Additive, or more than additive, effects from multiple exposures to an array of organic carcinogens in water are of such significance as to warrant an appraisal of the opportunity for magnification of the total carcinogenic burden which may be tractable or controllable by water processing to reduce the levels of total exposure.

4. The lack of a recognizable threshold for carcinogens implies that even a low level of exposure may contribute to the total cancer risk. Any reduction in the exposure to a carcinogen may, therefore, contribute to reducing the cancer risk in the general population.

5. The fact that some carcinogens from drinking water may persist in body tissues makes quantification of effects difficult.

6. Risks at defined exposure levels calculated for the carcinogens in drinking water emphasize the fact that there are finite risks from contaminants in drinking water.

Examples of changing regulations which demonstrate the flexibility of the system are shown nicely in the accompanying table from Morgan (1978) demonstrating recommended values for radiation exposure. An often discussed dichotomy can also be seen within this table since the occupationally exposed worker is allowed considerably more radiation than the general public. Such variation in exposure allowances is important in evaluating long-term effects and making extrapolations to risk hazards of the general public. The situation whereby the worker is allowed more heavy exposure than the general public is not an unusual circumstance.

Changes in Levels of Permissible Exposure to Ionizing Radiation

For Radiation Workers		For Members of the Public	
Recommended Values		Recommended Values	
1925: 0.1 erythema dose/y	52 R/y	1952: 0.03 rem/wk	1.5 rem/y
1934: 0.1 R/day (or 0.5 R/wk)	36 R/y	1959: 0.5 rem/y	0.5 rem/y
1949: 0.3 rem/wk	15 rem/y	1958: 5 rem/30 y	0.17 rem/y
1956: 5 rem/y	5 rem/y	1977: 25 mrem/y	0.025 rem/y
		1974: 5 mrem/y	0.005 rem/y

R — roentgen (1 R = 0.88 rem)
rem = roentgen equivalent man
mrem = millirem

Teratogenesis

Teratogenesis, most simply defined as the production
of birth defects, is an area of chemical toxicology which
is most often studied in experimental animals. Prior to
the marketing of any drug, the drug is subjected to a
series of tests in experimental animals whereby the animal being studied is given varying dosages of the compound beginning shortly after conception and then
carried on through most, if not all, of the gestational
period. The ability of a drug to produce a teratogenic
effect does not necessarily exclude it from public use.
There are many therapeutic drugs whose value is considered great enough to allow them to be available and, of
course, arbitrary limits of safety are always set. The
accompanying table compares therapeutic doses in animals
with the clinical dose given to human beings.

Chemical	Teratogenic Dose	Clinical Dose Per 24 Hrs.	Safety By Dose
Caffeine	75 mg/kg	2.5 mg/kg	30
Chlortetracycline	10 mg/kg	20.0 mg/kg	0.5
Diazepam	200 mg/kg	0.8 mg/kg	250
Phenytoin	75 mg/kg	6.0 mg/kg	12.5
Vitamin A	35,000 I.U.	8,000 I.U.	1,000 I.U.*
Prednisolone	2.5 mg/kg	0.2 mg/kg	125
Reserpine	1.5 mg/kg	0.02 mg/kg	75
Tetracycline	40 mg/kg	20 mg/kg	2
Salicylate	300 mg/kg	50 mg/kg	6

* adjusted to I.U./kg

The following table illustrates a number of those drugs
which are commonly used in clinical medicine which have
a demonstrated ability to produce a teratogenic effect.
   In studies with experimental animals, it is important
not only to give an adequate dose to produce a teratogenic effect and also to produce this effect without evidence of other toxicity to the animal, but also to produce
this effect through the period of development of the
embryo where the genetic apparatus is susceptible. The
exact point of this susceptibility, usually referred to
as the "window", is not known prior to the development of
a drug, although sometimes it can be predicted on the
basis of the chemical structure. Therefore, the drug is

Teratogens Used In Clinical Medicine

Chemical	Dosage
Acetazolamide	0.6% (in diet)
ACTH	5 mg q 6 h/3 days
Actinomycin D	25-100 mcg/kg
Alcohol	1.0-210 gm/kg
Aldosterone	0.05 mg/day
Amantadine HCl	10 mg/kg
Aminophyllin	100-200 mg/kg
Aminopterin	0.1 mg/kg
Anesthetics	-----
Antibodies	-----
Apomorphine	0.025 mg/embryo (chick)
Barbituric Acid	0.16% (mice) (in diet)
Busulfan	18-34 mg/kg
Caffeine	75-150 mg/kg
Chlorambucil	8-12 mg/kg
Chloramphenicol	100-200 mg/kg
Chlortetracycline	10 mg/kg
Colchicine	1-2 mg/kg (monkey)
Cortisone	-----
Coumarin Derivatives	4 mg/kg (mice)
Dextroamphetamine Sulfate	1 mg/kg
Diazepam	200 mg/kg
Diethylstilbestrol	10-42 mg
Dimethyl Sulfoxide	4.0 ml/kg
Diphenylhydantoin	75-150 mg/kg (mice)

Rat data unless otherwise noted

From Shepard (1976)

Teratogens Used In Clinical Medicine (cont'd)

Chemical	Dosage
Disulfiram	100 mg (in diet)
L–Dopa	10 mg/kg
Epinephrine	1–50 mcg
Fluorouracil	12–37 mg/kg
Griseofulvin	50–500 mg/kg
Hypervitaminosis A	35,000 I.U.
Imipramine	15 mg/kg
Isoniazid	-----
Lithium	212 mg/kg then 85 mg/kg
Marihuana	4.2 mg/kg
Meclizine	20–80 mg/kg
Methaqualone	0.8% (in diet)
Methotrexate	10 mg/kg (mice)
Nitrous Oxide	50% (by inhalation)
Noradrenalin	25 mcg/embryo
Phenobarbital	0.16% (mice) (in diet)
Physostigmine	0.05–15.0 mg/embryo (chick)
Pilocarpine	3–12 mg/embryo (chick)
Prednisolone	2.5 mg/kg
Prochlorperazine	2.5–10 mg/day
Reserpine	1.5 mg/kg
Salicylate	300 mg/kg
Sulphonamides	50 mg/kg
Tetracycline	40–80 mg/kg
Tolbutamide	300 mg/day

Rat data unless otherwise noted

From Shepard (1976)

given through most of the gestational period. Studies on
one mammal usually can be extrapolated to man in terms of
their effect since the teratogenic effect upon a rat is
commonly the same which will be produced in man. It is
important to remember that the drug must be given throughout the entire "window" period and that a single dosage
will not, in itself, produce the teratogenic effect even
though the teratogenic dose may be given at that time.
If a single dose is administered, this dose must be
larger than that which is established as the teratogenic
dose in experimental animals and the size of the single
dose is dependent upon such factors as metabolism, excretion and so forth.

In man, assessing the teratogenic effect of a chemical
in the environment is much more difficult than in the
experimental situation. Obviously, in the latter, many
variables can be held constant, whereas, this is certainly not true in human exposure situations. In humans, one
looks for evidence of increased rates of spontaneous
abortions, changes in neo-natal or peri-natal mortality,
changes in male:female ratio at birth, weight of newborns
or the production of congenital malformations. The most
important of these is probably the rate of spontaneous
abortions but the true rate of this phenomenon is not easy
to assess. Most spontaneous abortions occur in the first
trimester of pregnancy but most of these are not seen in
hospitals where accurate records are kept which can be
easily recalled for analysis. Rather, most spontaneous
abortions occur at home and only a percentage of these are
actually seen in physician's offices. Since abortions are
considered to occur prior to 20 weeks gestational age,
these statistics are not kept by the State Health Departments. Rather, what is reportable to Departments of
Vital Statistics is the incidence of fetal death, i.e.
death after 20 weeks gestation. The incidence of abortion under 20 weeks far outnumbers the incidence of fetal
deaths, therefore, vital statistics in this country are
not totally reliable and only give a general index of the
problem.

In addition to vital statistics, other sources for
assessing the problem of incidence of spontaneous abortion are available. Hospital records can be reviewed in
a retrospective manner but since only a small proportion,
as noted, of abortions appear in the hospitals, these
tend to underestimate the situation.

Retrospective surveys of selected population samples
can be performed but are open to question. In the WHO

Bulletin (1970) commenting on the problems of spontaneous
and induced abortions, it was noted that women interview-
ed in a nationwide survey in a country where abortion was
freely available only admitted to about half as many induced abortions as were known to have occurred by records
of therapeutic abortions which were already available.
Surveys can be performed of obstetric patients but the
weakness of this method is that it only includes abortions that are followed by another pregnancy. Conversely,
with regard to spontaneous abortions, a bias may be introduced whereby women who experience abortions are more
likely to undertake additional pregnancies than those who
carry their earlier pregnancies to term and this kind of
bias tends to increase the apparent incidence of spontaneous abortions among the population under study. Another possibility of distortion is introduced by the fact
that abortions tend to reoccur. Studies have been performed on the histories of gynecological patients, however, such histories are usually considered unreliable
and, in addition, pathological conditions which may have
caused a spontaneous abortion may not be remembered
after a period of years. In Family Planning Clinics,
studies on the rates of spontaneous abortions introduce
a double bias which tends to reduce the incidence of
spontaneous abortions and to increase the incidence of
induced abortions.

Prospective surveys have also been performed and in
these types of surveys, two methods are applied. One is
to identify a group of women and to periodically re-inter-
view them in order to determine the occurrence of pregnancies, births, and abortions during each interval. The
second method is to identify women as early as possible
in pregnancy and to follow them throughout the course in
order to identify the end results.

One thing which is very clear is that the general public is not aware that a spontaneous abortion is a fairly
frequent occurrence. The most singly important factor in
incidence of abortions appears to be the maternal age at
the time of conception. (Spouse age has never been studied although possibly it is also an important factor.)
In the woman of 19 years or under, the rate of spontaneous
abortion is about 10%. This rate then gradually increases
and by the age of 40, the rate of spontaneous abortions
is better than 33%. In addition, the above figures do not
include a number of spontaneous abortions which undoubtedly occur, based upon studies in experimental animals,
without any significant evidence to the mother that con-

ception has actually occurred. Such examples of early
abortions would include incomplete implantation of the
fertilized ovum occurring at a very early stage or incomplete transfer of the ovum to the uterus.

At the present time, it is believed that in the general
population, the incidence of spontaneous abortions is
somewhere in the range of 15-20%. Superimposed upon this
figure would be additional birth defects such as congenital malformations, neo-natal or peri-natal problems and
so forth.

One method of assessing the possibility of the etiology
of spontaneous abortions is to perform chromosome studies
upon fetal or embryonic tissue. This is, of course, a
difficult study to perform but at least it is known that
about 25% of spontaneously aborted conceptuses have
chromosomal defects compared with approximately 2.5% of
conceptuses obtained by induced (therapeutic) abortions.

Finally, it should be remembered that a variety of
factors other than chemicals may play a role in the development of spontaneous abortions. These include well
established genetic factors and infectious factors -
particularly viruses, immunological problems, anatomical
variations of either the mother or of the placenta and
the still unknown role of the male determinants.

Summary

The importance of the assessment of types, metabolism,
distribution, etc. and the effect upon the genetic make-
up of mankind is, obviously, a critical issue in the use
of chemicals in any industry. In order to safeguard our
future generations, as well as to avoid certain dilator-
ious effects upon the present, the importance of this
issue cannot be diminished. Although the potentially
harmful effects may be many years in the future, our
efforts to prevent such effects need to be taken in the
present. They likewise need to be taken with the best
scientific knowledge that we have available with the
recognition that certain changes in our thinking will
probably occur with the passage of time and, therefore,
the current regulations need to be flexible. The inability of scientists to clearly extrapolate experimental
evidence to man needs to be taken into consideration and
regulations must deal with this problem also in order to
avoid premature decisions. Eventually, the final
decision of safety will rest upon the shoulders of
society and not on any single group.

References

Ercegovich, C.D. and K.A. Rashid (1977) Mutagenesis
induced in mutant strains of Salmonella typhimurium
by pesticides. Amer Chem Soc Abstr Paper 174:Pest 43.

Hooper, N.K., R.H. Harris and B.A. Ames (1979) Chemical
carcinogens. Science 203:602-603.

Maugh, T.H. (1978) Chemical carcinogens: How dangerous
are low doses? Science 202:37-41.

McElheny, V.K. and S. Abrahamson (Eds.)(1979) Banbury
Report. 1. Assessing Chemical Mutagens: The Risk To
Humans, Cold Springs Harbor Laboratory, pp. 319-328.

Miller, E.C. and J.A. Miller (1979) Milestones in
chemical carcinogenesis. Sem Oncol 6:445-460.

Morgan, K.Z. (1978) Cancer and low level ionizing
radiation. Bull Atom Sci 34:30-41.

Neel, J.V. (1977) Monitoring for genetic effects in man.
IN: Environmental Monitoring, National Academy of
Sciences, Washington, DC, pp. 113-129.

Roberts, C.J. (1972) The effect of prolonged drug usage
on fetal development. An epidemiological approach.
IN: Drugs and Fetal Development, Klingberg, M.A.,
A. Abramovici and J. Chemke (Eds), Plenum Press,
New York, p. 457.

Trosko, J.E. and E.H.Y. Chu (1975) The role of DNA
repair and somatic mutation in carcinogenesis.
IN: Advances in Cancer Research, Klein, G. (Ed),
Academic Press, New York, 21:391-425.

Van Ryzin, J. (1980) Quantitative risk assessment.
J Occup Med 22:321-326.

Wahrendorf, J. (1979) The problem of estimating safe
dose levels in chemical carcinogenesis. J Cancer
Res Clin Oncol 95:101-107.

Warkany, J. (1972) Congenital Malformations through the
ages. IN: Drugs and Fetal Development, Klingberg
M.A., A. Abramovici and J. Chemke (Eds), Plenum Press
New York, pp. 7-15.

WHO Report (1970) Spontaneous and induced abortions.
    Wld Hlth Org Techn Rep Ser #461, pp 5-51.

Yerushalmy, J. (1972) Methodologic problems encountered
    in investigating the possible teratogenic effects of
    drugs. IN: Drugs and Fetal Development, Klingberg,
    M.A., A. Abramovici and J. Chemke (Eds), Plenum Press,
    New York, pp. 427-440.

Environmental Mutagen Society (Committee 17) (1975)
    Environmental Mutagenic Hazards. Science 187:503-514.

5

Regulatory Agencies

Introduction

Regulatory control of agricultural chemicals occurs
at all levels; county, state, and federal. At the federal level, the Environmental Protection Agency has the
major responsibility. Placed under this agency, the
1976 passage of the Toxic Substances Control Act was a
significant legislation since the Act shifted responsibility of testing for toxicity from government to
industry. The regulation of commercial chemicals is,
of course, a monumental task as there are currently an
estimated 70,000 types in use. The National Institute
of Occupational Safety and Health annually publishes a
Registry of Toxic Effects of Chemical Substances which
in 1978 contained about 34,000 entries. Inclusion on
this list, however, does not mean that the substance is
necessarily toxic to human beings, but only that the
substance has some evidence for toxicity. For example,
salt, a chemical required by the body, is included in
the registry.

The future role of the variety of agencies remains
open to question. Agencies are open to criticism from
all sides. They have been called a tax on innovation,
a means of spurring innovation, a means of forcing search
for substitutes, and, a means of controlling technology.
They have been accused of being simplistic, since once
legislation has been passed, the public may feel that
any crisis may be over, whereas nothing is probably
further from the truth. Indeed, it has been stated that
in some ways, when the law is passed, the crisis is just

beginning. Furthermore, legislation leads to the development of a superstructure of regulations which may be
built upon a weak scientific foundation. Indeed, our
regulatory process depends not only upon scientific, but
upon economic, social and medical foundations as well.
All these foundations may not be too firm.

The economics surrounding these chemicals is open to
debate. Although perhaps simplistic, society argues
whether one is distinguishing between freedom to versus
freedom from. The medical community is frequently not
aware of how to recognize environmental disease and,
indeed, there is even question about what are the criteria for these diseases. Setting standards is most
difficult, although by necessity it must be particularly
detailed, and the detail leads to a dependence upon
scientific technology or knowledge which is less than
perfect or complete.

Unfortunately, the regulatory agencies also inately
lead to the development of an adversary process. It
would probably be unusual if the Environmental Protection
Agency, as an example, were not being sued at the same
time and on the same issue by different groups taking
diametrically opposed positions.

The decisions reached by governmental regulatory
agencies are difficult ones. Input is from numerous
sources. In the case of the scientific viewpoint on
chemicals, the first step requires a knowledgeable scientific panel to review literature in order to reach some
opinion regarding safety from a toxicological standpoint.
Economic factors are currently a consideration and need
to be assessed in some manner through risk-benefit. The
public, either alone or through organized groups or its
elected representatives, can exert significant pressure
which may outweigh either scientific or economic issues.
Fortunately, the regulatory process does have some flexibility and is subject to change. For example, the
passage of the Occupational Safety and Health Act was
initially hailed by many as a great step forward in the
protection of workers. However, as multitudes of rules
and regulations began to be developed, the wisdom of
these regulations came under considerable criticism by
industry, and in late 1978, OSHA rescinded a number of
its previously published regulations under this law.
The regulatory agencies may also come under criticism
from other governmental agencies. For example, the
Environmental Protection Agency's recently proposed
changes in national ambient air quality standards for

photochemical oxidants (smog) came under heavy fire from
the Council on Wage and Price Stability (CWPS). The
CWPS criticized the EPA heavily stating that it did not
consider aggragate exposure to ozone nor did it provide
adequate rationale for its crucial policy choices in the
application of its methodology and had pushed the standards in a direction that was more stringent than necessary. The CWPS criticized the standard for ambient air
quality stating that the costs of meeting such new standards would range from $14.3-18.8 billion per year - as
opposed to the EPA estimate of $6.9-9.5 billion per year.
In either case, the CWPS felt that the marginal costs of
the newly proposed standards would be in the range of
$1100-4100 per reduced person-hour of ozone exposure and
felt that this was an unreasonable and inflationary
expenditure for a chemical which was only known to cause
a reversible discomfort and which apparently had no long-
term debilitating effects.

The difficulties of performing pesticide regulation
are demonstrated by assessing the problems of potential
carcinogens. This issue has been addressed by the Carcinogen Assessment Group of the Environmental Protection
Agency who conclude that risk-benefit ratio must be
considered in regulations. The problems for assessing
risk are well known and the problem of appraisal benefit
is difficult because there is not a straightforward
method for assessing this parameter and making comparison.
The Carcinogenic Assessment Group does not deny the
importance of experimental animal investigation but notes
that the methods of extrapolation from experimental data
to humans are also beset with multiple difficulties and
inaccuracies of assessment. Principal among this, particularly in addressing the problem of carcinogens, is
the pitfall which arises out of the large number of
experimental animals which must be used to practically
apply the data - even if one makes direct use of the
dose-response-nonthreshold approach.

The remainder of this section will discuss some of
the major environmental regulatory processes as well as
giving some of the more important addresses and telephone
numbers from which information may be sought regarding
environmental problems. This section is not, however,
intended to be a complete guide into the regulatory
system.

The RPAR Process

As a means of allowing issues of scientific question
and merit to be raised and discussed in a public manner,
the Federal Insecticide, Fungicide and Rodenticide Act
(FIFRA) developed a process referred to as the Rebuttable
Presumption Against Registration (RPAR). This process is
handled by the Special Pesticide Review Division, Office
of Pesticide Programs, Office of Pesticides and Toxic
Substances, EPA. Using certain definitions of risk criteria that, when met or exceeded, can trigger an RPAR
analysis, the chemical is reviewed extensively by a variety of scientists and published under an RPAR document.
The risk criteria, originally published in the Federal
Register on July 3, 1975 (40CFR162.11), are concerned
with the following areas:

1. Acute toxicity
2. Chronic toxicity
   a. oncogenic
   b. mutagenic
3. Other chronic effects
   a. reproductive
      1) fetotoxicity
      2) teratogenicity
   b. spermatogenicity
   c. testicular effects
4. Significant reduction in wildlife, reduction in a
   dangerous species and reduction in non-target
   species
5. Lack of emergency treatment or antidote

Presently, the Office of Pesticide Programs (OPP) in
the EPA is facing the task of which chemicals, numbering
in the thousands, to look at and regulate first. This
is not easy since much information which is needed for
decision making is far from complete. Because of the
lack of a sufficiently designed internal system for
identifying and ranking chemicals which might come under
the cost-benefit assessment procedure or the Rebuttable
Presumption Against Registration (RPAR), a system has
been suggested whereby the OPP would be able to apply
some formal procedure and assessment of a limited number
of chemicals based upon three categories. The first
category would be the apparently dangerous compounds
which would be scheduled for review in accordance with
the urgency of the situation, whereby urgency is a

function of toxic potency and the extent of exposure.
Compounds for which there are insufficient data to make
a determination should be those next scheduled for additional study, with those compounds involved in the
greatest exposure receiving the earliest attention and
then, based upon the further studies, the decision might
be made whether the chemical belongs under the RPAR
system. Finally, the third class compounds would be
those in which there is no evidence to suspect that a
material is hazardous when used as directed and these
would simply be re-registered without any further consideration.

In continuing the above procedure, it is assumed that
the classes of compounds either apparently dangerous or
those with insufficient data present would be disallowed
immediately if risks were greater than benefits in an
obvious manner. If substitutes were available and risks
were greater than benefits, then RPAR evaluation would
be instigated.

The above method for recommending and selecting pesticide formulations for registration does definitely take
into assessment the risk-benefit of chemicals toward
society. The method of observing or assessing the empirical data on mutagenic, teratogenic or carcinogenic
effects of the pesticides is still a difficult procedure
and the basis for inferring these effects from laboratory
experiments is not always complete. Nevertheless, estimates are made, but it is currently recommended that the
new assessments of the incidence of human diseases, such
as cancer, should not be used in the decision-making
process until our understanding of the mechanisms of
cancer permits us to draw more reliable numerical extrapolation to humans from the kind of laboratory data
which is currently available.

The RPAR is divided into a variety of categories.
The first of these is the Pre-RPAR. This is simply an
initial risk investigation phase that involves a scientific review of studies in the literature to evaluate
whether RPAR criteria have been exceeded by the chemical
which is being questioned. If such a "trigger study"
suggests that an RPAR criterion is being exceeded, the
Agency then extrapolates from models or known information
and attempts to develop "worst case" exposure assumptions
and to hypothesize the potential risk of the pesticide
under review. The literature search put together by the
investigative team with the combination of the hazard
information regarding risk exposure is then published in

the form of a document describing the position on risk and referred to as Position Document 1 (PD1). The PD1 is then published in the Federal Register along with a formal notice of presumption against registration.

After the PD1 is published, the public process begins and a 45 day period is allowed for comment on the PD1, in addition to a 60 day extension, if justified. Therefore, technically there may be an 105 day period from the time the PD1 is published to the Agency's initial action. Testimony may be submitted by any interested parties. If all the "triggers" have been successfully rebutted in the opinion of the Agency, the pesticide is returned to the registration process and the RPAR is terminated for either all or some of its uses. At this time, a second position document (PD2) is drafted which states the Agency's regulatory action for the chemical. The Agency only publishes a separate PD2 in those cases where the rebuttal has been successful. When rebuttal is not successful, rebuttal assessment, risk analysys, benefit analysis, etc., and the proposed regulatory changes or position are presented in a document called the PD2/3. The latter consists of 1) an introductory chapter reviewing the RPAR criteria giving rise to the review, 2) the Risk Analysis, the Benefit Analysis, the risk/benefit analysis or ratio, and 4) the recommended regulatory position. The PD2/3 is then published in the Federal Register. At this point, the FIFRA requires that the proposed regulatory decision be submitted to a Scientific Advisory Panel (SAP) for review of the scientific basis of the proposed decision, as well as to the Secretary of Agriculture for comment. These comments, plus any other industry or public comments, are then again evaluated and the final regulatory decision is published in the Federal Register under the heading of the PD4. As of July 1980, the following chemicals had received RPAR status.

Chemicals on RPAR - 1980

2,4,5-T
Diallate
Ethylene dibromide
Pronamide
Toxaphene
Thiophanate-methyl
Pentachloronitrobenzene (PCNB)
Dibromochloropropane (DBCP)

Maleic hydrazide
Ethylenebisdithiocarbamates
Amitraz
Cadmium
Ethylene oxide
Kepon (Chlordecone)
Dimethoate
Endrin
Benomyl
Strychnine
Strychnine sulfate
Compound 1080 (sodium fluoroacetate)
Compound 1081 (fluroacetamide)

Once a chemical has been placed on the RPAR list, the registrant of that chemical assumes the burden of proof that the chemical is not a risk and should continue in use. Three methods of proof are available.

1) In the case of a chemical which has been questioned because of its possible acute toxicity problems, the registrant must prove that the chemical will not be acutely toxic to the applicator or to the overall population of both the target and non-target organisms when the chemical is used under the proper methods.

2) In the case of a chemical which is presumed to be toxic for chronic problems, the registrant must prove that under normal methods of use, the pesticide will not concentrate, persist or accrue in man or the environment at levels which are likely to result in any of the addressed chronic adverse effects.

3) In either case, that is, either acute or chronic, the registrant may also attempt to prove that the chemical does not meet or exceed any of the known criteria for risk.

The registrant also has the option, in addition to submitting evidence in order to rebut the presumption of an acute or chronic risk, of submitting evidence that the economic, social or environmental benefits from the continued use of the chemical under question will outweigh the risk of use. In this case, if the risk presumptions are not rebutted, the benefit evidence submitted may then be taken into account and if it can be determined that benefits do, indeed, outweigh risk, the chemical may continue to be utilized. At any time that the regulatory agency determines that an "imminent hazard" exists for either humans or the environment, the chemical may be suspended from all further use. The difficulty of interpretation is obviously what criteria are used to determine benefit versus risk and also what is the definition of "imminent hazard". As an example of a difficult problem, determining "imminent hazard" with a mutagenic compound is, in reality, an impossibility since the effect will not be seen for years. Therefore, regulatory agencies must rely upon current scientific methods plus interpretation - which are sometimes argumentative - in order to assess the possibility of hazard.

For those interested in knowing the status report and where to get material on Rebuttable Presumption Against Registration and registration standards, the following office should be written to:

> Office of Pesticides Program (TS-791)
> U.S. Environmental Protection Agency
> 401 "M" Street S.W.
> Washington, DC 20460

Toxic Substances Control Act

The Toxic Substances Control Act (TSCA) is a federal legislation which was enacted by Congress in 1976 and became effective in January of 1977, at the beginning of President Carter's term. President Nixon is cited as promoting the initial concept for legislation in his speech to Congress in February of 1971 with the concern that steps needed to be taken to prevent chemicals from becoming environmental hazards. Legislation was gradually developed with the general idea of having a system of pre-marketing notification and testing so that the thousands of chemicals which are regularly introduced into commerce would have adequate testing prior to their introduction into the environment. The intent of the law is to protect human health, however, the actual testing is directed principally at the health effects, such as oncogenicity, teratogenicity, mutagenicity and environmental fate, persistence and ecological effects. The legal machinery for this organization is under the control of the Environmental Protection Agency. Inven-

tories are updated regularly and in July of 1980, there
were a total of more than 55,000 chemicals which were
subject to the TSCA. The principal mechanism of evaluation, however, is still through the pre-manufacturing
notification (PMN) requirements which must be followed
prior to the introduction of a chemical by any manufacturer into the commercial market.

Notifications are published on a regular basis through
the TSCA Chemicals in Progress Bulletin and administered
through the EPA Office of Pesticides and Toxic Substances
in Washington, DC.

Threshold Limit Values

The American Conference of Governmental Industrial
Hygienists annually publishes a booklet entitled, "Thresh-
hold Limit Values For Chemical Substances in Workroom
Air". This booklet is an actual listing of a number of
chemicals and the recommended threshold limit values
(TLV) for safeguarding the worker. These recommendations
have a scientific basis, which is published in a separate
booklet. Both of these booklets may be obtained from the
American Conference of Governmental Industrial Hygienists
(ACGIH) at P.O. Box 1937, Cincinnati, OH 45201.

The TLVs refer to working conditions, principally
airborne, which workers may be exposed to repeatedly on
a daily basis. The ACGIH points out specifically that it
does not have any legal, i.e. regulatory, strength in
developing these TLVs. Furthermore, the TLVs are sometimes overly interpreted. The authors of the TLV booklets point out specifically that there may be a wide
variation in individual susceptibility and, therefore,
a small percentage of workers may experience some discomfort at the TLVs which are published. Furthermore, a
wide variety of TLVs actually exist. They are:

1) The Threshold Limit Value - Time Weighted Average
(TLV-TWA) - ths is the time weighted average of concentration for a normal eight hour workday or 40 hour work
week, to which nearly all workers may be repeatedly exposed, day after day, without adverse effect.

2) The Threshold Limit Value - Short-Term Exposure
Limit (TLV-STL) - this is the maximum concentration to
which workers may be exposed for a period of up to 15
minutes continuously without expecting to suffer any ill
effects.

3) The Threshold Limit Value - Ceiling (TLV-C) - this
is the concentration that should not be exceeded even
instantaneously.

Again, the ACGIH points out that the TLVs are guidelines and are not meant as absolute figures. The limits
are intended principally for the use of industrial hygienists or other individuals who are trained in this discipline or in occupational medicine. The TLVs are not
intended for use as a relative index of hazard or toxicity, the evaluation or control of community air pollution instances, estimating the toxic potential of work
exposure, as proof or disproof of an existing disease or
physical condition, or for adoption by countries other
than the United States where processes or substances may
differ from the work practices in the United States.
    In spite of the above caveats, the threshold limit
values are used regularly by industry and are referred
to as a guideline for safe work practices. A number of
agricultural chemicals are also listed by the ACGIH as
having threshold limit values.

Federal Agencies

    A number of federal offices exist that can be con-
tacted for information regarding not only the regulations
for agricultural chemicals, but for other information
regarding basic toxicology or use. They are listed below.

EPA	NIOSH	OSHA
1200 Sixth Avenue	Arcade Building	1808 Smith Tower
Seattle, WA 98101	1321 Second Ave.	506 Second Avenue
(206) 442-1090	Seattle, WA 98101	Seattle, WA 98104
	(206) 442-0530	(206) 442-5930

The following federal agencies are coordinating efforts
to protect rural workers and communities from pesticide
poisoning.

EPA

Assistant Administrator for
Pesticides and Toxic Substances
401 M Street S.W.
Washington, DC 20460

U.S. Department of Health and Human Services

Deputy Director
Office of Primary Care
5600 Fishers Lane
Rockville, MD 20857

U.S. Department of Labor

Office of Program Development and
    Accountability
Employment Standards Administration
200 Constitution Avenue N.W.
Washington, DC 20210

National Migrant Labor Coordinator
Occupational Safety and Health
    Administration

U.S. Department of Education

Division of Migrant Education
400 Maryland Avenue S.W.
Washington, DC 20202

U.S. Department of Agriculture

Office of Environmental Quality
14th & Independence Ave. S.W.
Washington, DC 20250

Community Services Administration

1200 - 19th Street N.W.
Washington, DC 20036

Pacific Northwest Agencies

Idaho

Department of Agriculture
P.O. Box 790
Boise, ID 83701
(208) 334-3242

OSHA
1315 W. Idaho Street
Boise, ID 83707
(208) 342-1867

Department of Public Health
State House
Boise, ID 83720
(208) 334-3401

Oregon

Department of Agriculture
Agriculture Building
Salem, OR 97310
(503) 378-4665

OSHA
New Federal Building
Suite 640
1220 S.W. Third Avenue
Portland, OR 97204
(503) 221-2251

Department of Human Resources
Health Division
1400 S.W. Fifth Avenue
Portland, OR 97201
(503) 229-5910

Washington

Department of Agriculture
General Administration Bldg.
P.O. Box 128
Olympia, WA 98501
(206) 753-5050

OSHA
121 - 107th Avenue N.E.
Bellevue, WA 98004
(206) 442-7520

Health Services Division
P.O. Box 1788
Olympia, WA 98504
(206) 753-5871

Acronyms of Commonly Encountered Federal Agencies

A number of agencies at the federal level are responsible for the regulation of chemicals. Frequently, they
are referred to by their acronyms rather than their full
names. These acronyms with their full name follow:

CEQ   - Council on Environmental Quality
EPA   - Environmental Protection Agency
FDA   - Food and Drug Administration
FIFRA - Federal Insecticide, Fungicide and Rodenticide
        Act
GAO   - General Accounting Office
HHS   - Health and Human Services Department
        (formerly Health, Education and Welfare)
IRLG - Interagency Regulatory Liaison Group
ITC   - TSCA Interagency Testing Committee
NTP   - National Toxicology Program, HHS
OECB - Organization for Economic Cooperation and
        Development
OMB   - Office of Management and Budget
OPTS - Office of Pesticides and Toxic Substances,
        including
        OPP - Office of Pesticide Programs
        OTS - Office of Toxic Substances
OSHA - Occupational Safety and Health Administration
OSW   - Office of Solid Waste, EPA
PTSED - Pesticide and Toxic Substances Enforcement
        Division, EPA
RCRA - Resource Conservation and Recovery Act
RPAR - Rebuttable Presumption Against Registration
        (pesticides)
TSCA - Toxic Substances Control Act
USDA - U.S. Department of Agriculture

Summary

What can be expected in the next three to five decades
regarding the current trends of chemical use and their
likely impact upon environmental problems? The problem
is a vexing one. It has been addressed by many people
and is currently addressed by increasing numbers of both
the public and scientists. Recently, the National Academy of Sciences convened in a workshop under the chair-
manship of Dr. John Cantlon (1979), to specifically
address these issues. A number of examples of future
trends were cited.

1) It is anticipated that there will be a gradual
reduction in the large backlog of chemical compounds for
which adequate risk information is lacking. This backlog
will diminish both as research information becomes more
available and as certain "problem" compounds are with-
drawn from the U.S. markets. It is likely that there
will be fewer new chemicals which lack adequate assessment of their potential impact on the environment as
current techniques of toxicological assessment are brought
into use for all the new chemicals. The latter will
probably lead to the reduction of small companies who
are currently marketing some compounds and will strengthen
the market for large industry.

2) As inflation and the price of energy continue to
push upward, many marginal chemicals currently in pro-
ductive use will probably leave the market.

3) New technologies should avoid many of the environmental problems by altered processes, providing that the
cost does not totally remove some chemicals completely
from the marketplace.

4) Expected improvements in containment and clean-up
procedures should alleviate some problems of hazards of
existing dump sites of chemicals and further regulations
would lead to more recycling or some form of destruction.

5) A growing scientific understanding will have to
develop of the impact of the mixtures of toxic substances
- such things as co-factors, inhibitors, synergisms or
interferences - and these should provide the public with
better knowledge of the risks from toxic chemicals.

6) Data bases, research models, training and data processing in human epidemiology and particularly in those aspects of clinical epidemiology should provide a firmer base for decision makers, researchers and for the public's understanding.

7) Industry will pay more attention to end-use risk assessment and will, therefore, design products with better instructions to users and disposal requirements.

8) The trade-offs between environmental improvements and the marketplace will become more apparent and market forces will be brought to bear on this type of assessment.

9) The public may show increasing concern for improving U.S. production to allow this country to compete more effectively in world trade and this will bring important environmental and occupational safety issues into sharp focus.

10) It is possiblt that growing public sophistication in toxicology, or with environmental concern, may ameliorate demands for zero risk technologies.

11) Continued experience between federal, state, local and industry representatives may bring better articulation among these groups and lead to decreased risk and improved environmental protection efforts.

12) It should be recognized that there will be growing pressure from the world's population on the earth's resources for energy, raw materials, water and food and that this pressure is liable to lead to increased use of polluting technologies, or at least the demand for such technologies, without waiting for very sophisticated testing or replacement methods. It is likely that, at least in developing countries, the problems of poverty, hunger, poor public health, poor communication and poor transportation will all lead to considerably more mortality and morbidity than polluting technologies.

13) It is hoped that improved scientific understanding of the effects of toxic materials on human health and behavior will lower the threshold for some materials, i.e. that improved understanding may alleviate some of the problems of concern at this time because of uncertainty regarding thresholds.

14) Improved instrumentation and data handling should provide a clearer picture of the extent of the chemicals in our society, therefore leading to better assessment of risk, including subtle effects upon humans, animals and plants.

15) Improvement in our knowledge about eco-systems will lead to better species or models of testing for environmental impact in experimental situations. On the other hand, better data may also create difficulties which occur beyond the national boundaries and this may lead to international problems whose resolutions are more difficult. Better information on unsafe use of hazardous materials will be made available to the general public and may indicate a larger risk than sometimes currently acknowledged.

16) Improvement in the technical biochemical procedures for analyzing human tissue may show that there is a wider population of human beings and animals with some degree of chemical contamination than is currently recognized.

17) Growing public concern in the United States about such things as the nation's defense capability, its trade deficit, and global economic recession will continue to have an impact and a considerable influence upon Congress, the courts and the general public, requiring, and perhaps making it difficult to pursue, what might be considered environmental improvements without very strong data which validate the serious effects from bona fide environmental hazards.

References

Cantlon, J. (Chrm) (1979) Long-Range Environmental Outlook. Proceedings of a Workshop, Environmental Studies Board: Commission on Natural Resources, National Research Council, National Academy of Sciences, November 14-16.

Part II
Individual Chemicals

Introduction

Part I of this book is an overview of the basic sciences necessary to understanding the use of agricultural chemicals. It also deals with some of the principal socio-economic issues. Part II of this book deals with the basic and clinical toxicology of selected agricultural chemicals as they are classified into different types of chemical structures. Unless one resorts to simplified tables or, alternatively, becomes excessively redundant, the large numbers of agricultural chemicals necessitate that this discussion be handled in such groups. This approach is used not only because of the large numbers of chemicals but because the manifestations of toxicity are often very similar within each class. Thus, the toxicity of the phenoxy herbicides would generally be the same whether discussing 2,4-D, 2,4,5-T or any of their esters. Similarly, treatment will generally be the same. When dealing with an agricultural chemical and uncertain about its toxicity, by identifying the basic chemical structure and classifying it, one can begin to make some basic assumptions regarding its clinical toxicity. The more known about the basic toxicology, the greater will be the predicitive accuracy of the clinical toxicology.

In each chapter of Part II, an attempt has been made to divide the discussion into sections on the basic chemistry, basic toxicology, molecular biology issues, environmental fate, potential human exposure, symptoms and signs of intoxication, and diagnosis and treatment. In the first categories, other texts are available for much more detail. For example, Audus (1976) is a detailed discussion on the physiology and biochemistry of the mechanism of herbicides. Several good references on the toxicology of pesticides exist, such as the text by

Hayes (1975) and the text by Matsumura (1975). For
details of organophosphate biochemistry and mechanism
of action, the text by Eto (1979) is useful. The Herbicide Handbook of the Weed Sciences Society of America
is annually updated and is an excellent source for basic
toxicology information and uses. Several large chemical
companies have a toll-free information line.

Worker Protection

    It would be desirable to never have any type of intox-
ication syndrome occur with any chemical. Worker protection is, of course, the basis for preventing most problems
which conceivably could occur. Protection varies with
individual chemicals and details of worker protection can
be obtained through the Agricultural Extension Services,
through the labels of chemicals, and through the local
OSHA offices. Workers should be educated about the
necessary self-care to prevent intoxication and both the
employer and employee should be held responsible for
safety in the field.
    In certain instances, it would seem advisable to not
allow people to work with these chemicals. Pre-employment screening, although not commonly performed, could
weed out individuals more likely to develop problems.
For example, with those persons who have pre-existing
neurological disease, it seems foolhardy for them to work
with organophosphates which might cause further neuropathy. Individuals with pre-existing hepatitis or chronic renal disease of any sort will have increased difficulty in the major metabolic mechanisms of detoxification
and excretion and therefore their risk will be increased.
Persons working with organophosphates on a regular basis
should routinely have blood cholinesterase levels performed. In addition, however, they should also have a
blood cholinesterase level performed prior to employment.
Those persons with any type of skin disease will certainly be more susceptible to absorption of chemicals and
therefore more prone to develop an intoxication syndrome.

Informational Sources

    Physicians are always aware of their local Poison
Control Center telephone number of some similar informational source. In dealing with agricultural chemicals,

they should also become familiar with the name of their
local Agricultural Extension agent and also be aware
that informational sources exist through the State Departments of Agriculture. The Agricultural Extension agent
is usually local and is frequently the only individual
who has a good knowledge of what chemicals are being used
within a particular county, how they are being applied,
when they are being applied, and by whom.

Sampling Procedures

   In all cases of suspected intoxication, it is critical
that both environmental samples as well as human tissue
samples such as blood or urine be taken and that the
diagnosis be substantiated rather than be simply alluded
to or assumed. Every attempt should be made to bring
symptoms and signs into the parameter of objective measurements through clinical biochemistry and including such
ancillary measures as nerve conduction studies, electro-
encephalograms, electrocardiograms and so forth when they
are indicated. In this age, biological samples can be
analyzed for almost any chemical which an individual has
been exposed to. Exposure must be documented. It is
therefore critical that the physician know the exact
chemical which is under suspicion. A copy of the label
is very helpful and the vehicle should be determined.
When uncertain of a diagnosis or when one wants to keep
the possibility of an intoxication syndrome as part of a
differential diagnosis, one should simply store urine and
serum in a frozen state until ready for some future
analysis. The practice of saving tissue samples at the
time of entrance into an Emergency Department is one
which can only be beneficial to the patient. It is also
the time when tissue levels will be at their highest.
   When obtaining and shipping samples for pesticide
residue analysis, it is helpful to call the performing
laboratory for information related to such procedures.
In Oregon, one should call the laboratory services at the
Department of Agriculture (telephone 378-3793). Samples
should be identified properly and contain information
such as sample type, location or tissue from which sample
was taken, date and time taken, the name of the party
requesting the sample and the type of analysis requested.
Samples are not always stable and should be shipped as
rapidly as possible. Refrigeration or frozen storage is
normally not required if the samples are sent within one

to three days, with the exceptions being perishable tissues or samples which contain highly volatile compounds such as Sevin. In the case of sample analysis for Roundup or Krenite, samples should also be refrigerated.

Avoidance of cross contamination of samples is important. Thus, sample collectors should be cautious in the handling of sampling jars and the possibility of contaminating their hands in the process of sample collection. The sampling specimen containers may or may not require some type of preservative. This is dependent upon the residue analysis being desired as well as the type of sample which is being shipped.

Confusion occasionally exists in the public's eye because of the way results, including the lower limits of detection, are reported. The detection limit (lower limit of detection) is that point at which there is no indication of any pesticide residue whatsoever. Levels below the detection limit may be recorded as equal to or less than the lower limit of detection or as "no residue". The confirmation limit is that point above which there is sufficient pesticide residue to assure its exact identity. This point is always higher than the detection limit. The no confirmable residue are those results between detection and confirmation limits. Samples with pesticide residues above the confirmation level are the actual levels reported. Samples below this level will frequently be reported with a sign as follows " $\leqq$ ". The distinction between these types of results should be kept clearly in mind as it is not unusual to have detection and confirmation levels confused with the misunderstanding that levels reported at the $\leqq$ or below the confirmable level actually exist rather than only being suspected or not at all present.

The sample size is dependent upon the material which is to be analyzed. In the case of clinical samples, the samples should always be taken under the supervision of a licensed physician or licensed clinical laboratory. In the case of blood analysis, 10 ml of blood should be submitted. Usually it is preferred in a heparinized form with the plasma and cells separated. In the case of urine, a sample of at least 200 cc's should be sent. If one desires a 24 hour excretion pattent, then, of course, one must submit a representation of a 24 hour sample (aliquot).

In the case of environmental sampling, most laboratories would prefer the following:

Sample Type	Recommended Minimum Amount
Water	1 gallon
Foliage	1-2 pounds
Soil	2-5 pounds
Tissue (whole fish, birds, small mammals, muscle portions of deer, elk, etc.)	1 pound

As in the case of sampling of human tissue, the sampling of environmental residues may be difficult and subject to numerous errors. Therefore, it is advisable to receive help from one of the State Departments of Agriculture regarding the correct manner of sampling material such as water, soil and so forth.

References

Audus, L.J. (Ed.)(1976) Herbicides, Academic Press, London.

Eto, M. (1979) Organophosphorus Pesticides: Organic and Biological Chemistry, CRC Press, Boca Raton, Florida.

Hayes, W.J.,Jr. (1975) Toxicology of Pesticides, The Williams & Wilkins Company, Baltimore.

Matsumura, F. (1975) Toxicology of Insecticides, Plenum Press, New York.

1

Pentachlorophenol

Pentachlorophenol is one of the most widely used pesticides in this country. It is used as an insecticide,
fungicide, herbicide, algacide, disinfectant, and as an
ingredient in antifouling paint. It finds applications
in industries manufacturing leather, masonry, wood and
wood products, cooling towers, rope, and paper mills.
The variety of trade names are as follows: Chem-Penta,
Chemtrol, Chlorophen, Dowicide EC-7, Dowicide G, Durotox,
Lauxtol A, Na-PCP, PCP, Penchlorol, Penta, Penta-kil,
Pentanol, Pentasol, Permacide, Permaguard, Permasem,
Permatox, Sinituho, Term-1-trol, Noxtane, and Weed-Beads.
The large majority of pentachlorophenol is then used
in the treatment of wood products, primarily as a fungicide and bacteriocide. It may be used in water systems
to control algae and fungi. In construction materials,
it may be found in tiles, shingles, concrete, asbestos,
pressboard and wallboard and insulation. It is used in
leather to prevent deterioration during tanning. In
paint, it can be used as a preservative. In the textile
industry, it prevents processed materials from developing
mildew. The chemical may come in contact with food since
its applications include its use in paper, adhesives,
plastics and so forth which would come in contact with
either the dry or aqueous food after packaging. In
short, the compound can be found in a wide variety of
places. It is estimated that the Pacific Northwest uses
5.5 million pounds per year.

Manufacture

The chemical is produced by the chlorination of molton phenol in a two-stage process. In the first stage, chlorination occurs producing analogs of tri- and tetrachlorophenol. In the second stage, the temperature is decreased slightly from the initial 105°C and the tri- and tetrachlorophenols are then further chlorinated to form pentachlorophenol. The chlorination action is not complete and tetrachlorophenols persist following the reaction such that technical grade pentachlorophenol contains 4-12% tetrachlorophenols.

The manufacture of any chlorophenol formulation can be expected to have a variety of impurities and this is true regardless of the nature of the final product, i.e. trichlorophenol, tetrachlorophenol, pentachlorophenol, etc. The principal impurities found are the pre-dioxins, dibenzofurans and a variety of chlorinated dioxins. A number of analogs also occur as the compounds are manufactured with the starting process occurring with phenol. These are demonstrated below.

Analogs manufactured by direct chlorination

2,4-Dichlorophenol   2,4,6-Trichloro-phenol   2,3,4,6-Tetra-chlorophenol   Pentachloro-phenol

The amount of impurities varies considerably but figures cited for formulations used as fungicides are:

Chlorinated dioxins	<1 —	2000 ppm
Chlorinated diphenylethers	100 —	1000 ppm
Chlorinated dibenzofurans	50 —	200 ppm
Chlorinated phenoxyphenols	~1%	

Examples of the chemical structure of the impurities
are shown below. A concern is that burning of chlorinated phenoxy phenols will yield chlorinated dioxins.
From the environmental standpoint, the thermal ring clos-
ure which occurs with burning can, therefore, potentially
lead to the production of a variety of chlorinated dioxins when sawdust or other sawmill waste which is contaminated with chlorophenols is burned and the effluent
passed into the atmosphere.

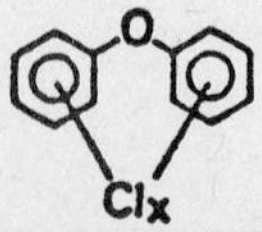

Diphenylethers

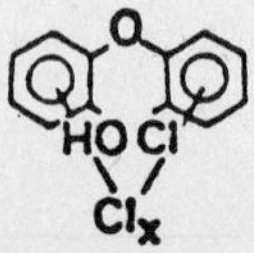

Predioxins

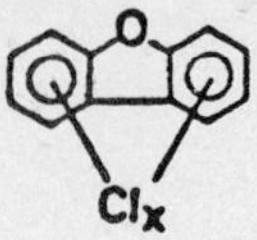

PCDFs

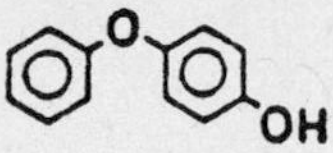

Isopredioxins

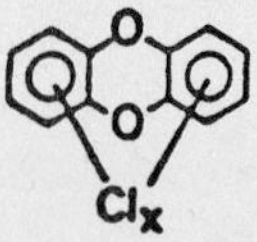

PCDDs

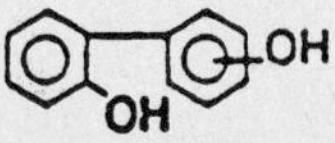

Di-OH PCB

Dioxin Contamination: Pentachlorophenol is contaminated with a variety of dioxins, principally the hexa-
chloro-, heptachloro-, and the octachlorodibenzo-p-dioxins
plus a variety of polychlorodibenzofurans. The most
definitive study of this nature has been reported by
Buser (1976a) and is summarized below.

Chlorodioxins and Chlorofurans in Dow PCP Products

Samples	PCDD(a) ppm			PCDF(b) ppm				
	Hexa-	Hepta-	Octa-	Tetra-	Penta-	Hexa-	Hepta-	Octa-
PCP (EC-7)	0.15	1.1	5.5	0.45	0.03	0.3	0.5	0.2
PCP (EC-7)	0.03	0.6	8.0	<0.02	<0.03	<0.03	<0.1	<0.1
PCP(c)	9.5	125	160	<0.02	0.05	15	95	105
PCP(c)	9.1	180	280	0.05	0.25	36	320	210
PCP-Na(c)	3.4	40	115	<0.02	0.05	11	50	24
PCP	10.0	130	210	0.20	0.20	13	70	55
PCP	5.4	130	370	0.07	0.20	9	60	65

(a) PCDD = Polychlorodibenzo-p-dioxin
(b) PCDF = Polychlorodibenzofuran
(c) Dow product, supplied by Fluka, a laboratory chemical supplier.

A study by Buser and Bosshardt (1976b) also demonstrated tetra-chlorinated dioxins in some commercial
samples. However, the 2,3,7,8-chlorine isomer was definitely not present.

It is clear that the concentrations of contaminating
dioxins vary depending upon the care of manufacture.
Examples of the differences in contaminating dioxins are
shown in the accompanying table by Crummett (1973).

Hexa- and Octachlorodioxins in Domestic PCPs

Sample	Mfgr	Hexachlorodioxin ppm[a]	Octachlorodioxin ppm[b]
1	Vulcan	10	1700
2	"	N.D.	N.D.
3	"	15	2500
4	"	16	3600
5	Reichhold	20	700
6	"	17	600
7	"	23	900
8	"	N.D.	N.D.
9	Monsanto	15	1400
10	"	12	1100
11	"	15	1900
12	Dow	N.D.	2
13	"	N.D.	2
14	"	N.D.	N.D.
15	"	16	1500
16	"	16	1800
17	"	21	3400

(a)   Detection limit 0.3 ppm, except for sample 8 which
      is 2 ppm; N.D. = not detected.
(b)   Detection limit 1 ppm, except for sample 8 which is
      6 ppm; N.D. = not detected.

Technical PCP contains contaminants other than dioxin,
among them are traces of trichlorophenol, chlorinated
dibenzofurans, chlorophenoxyphenols, chlorodiphenyl
ethers, chlorohydroxydiphenyl ethers, and traces of other
more complex reaction products of phenol.

An example of the ability to improve the quality of
commercial PCP is shown in the accompanying table illustrating first, the composition of commercial PCP under
usual manufacturing conditions and then the reduction of
contaminants by distillation in the second table.

Composition of a Commercial PCP
(Dowicide 7, Sample 9522 A)

Component	Analytical Results
Pentachlorophenol	88.4%
Tetrachlorophenol	4.4%
Trichlorophenol	< 0.1%
Chlorinated Phenoxyphenols	< 6.2%
Octachlorodioxin	2500 ppm
Heptachlorodioxins	125 ppm
Hexachlorodioxins	4 ppm
Octachlorodibenzofurans	80 ppm
Heptachlorodibenzofurans	80 ppm
Hexachlorodibenzofurans	30 ppm

Composition of Purified Grade PCP
(Dowicide EC-7)

Component	Analytical Results
Pentachlorophenol	89.8%
Tetrachlorophenol	10.1%
Trichlorophenol	< 0.1%
Octachlorodioxin	15.0 ppm
Heptachlorodioxins	6.5 ppm
Hexachlorodioxins	1.0 ppm
Octachlorodibenzofurans	< 1 ppm
Heptachlorodibenzofurans	1.8 ppm
Hexachlorodibenzofurans	< 1 ppm

Physical Properties

A summary of the physical properties of pentachlorophenol is shown in the table below. The product marketed
as a sodium salt has a high water solubility and therefore could be expected to have more mobility in the environment than the contaminating dioxins or dibenzofurans.

Properties of Pentachlorophenol (PCP)

Molecular Weight	266.35
Melting Point	$191^{\circ}C$
Boiling Point	$310^{\circ}C$ (decomposes)
Density	1.987
Vapor Pressure	1.6×10^{-4} mm Hg ($25^{\circ}C$)
	1.2×10^{-1} mm Hg ($100^{\circ}C$)
	40 mm Hg ($211^{\circ}C$)
Solubility H_2O	20 ppm at $30^{\circ}C$
Solubility of sodium salt, H_2O	33g/100g
Partition Coefficient	$1 \times 10^{5.01}$
Molar Refraction	53.5

The physical characteristics of the chemical allow for it to be found in a number of different environmental samples. PCP has been found in house dust, air and water and its presence in non-biological samples is probably explained by proximity to a source of PCP. The material can be taken into biological organisms by all three routes of exposure. The environmental distribution of the contaminating dioxins and dibenzofurans in the environment is less well known although the physical characteristics of the latter chemicals strongly suggest that these chemicals would not be widely distributed from the source. When pentachlorophenol is burned, it is transformed into dioxins, including the four chlorine form but not in high amounts or the most toxic 2,3,7,8-chlorodioxin according to Ahling and Johansson (1977).

Pentachlorophenol, as a free phenol, is absorbed readily on many surfaces, particularly soil. The sodium salt is also readily absorbed by suspended particulate matter, at least in water. PCP is susceptible to photochemical degradation in water and various solvents.

Animal Toxicology Studies

Oral: The LD_{50} for PCP by oral ingestion in male rats has been variously reported as ranging from 78 mg/kg to 205 mg/kg. For the female rat, the LD_{50} varys from 135 mg/kg to 175 mg/kg. The LD_{50} for mice was reported as 130 mg/kg; 130 mg/kg for rabbits; 250 mg/kg for guinea pigs; 120 mg/kg for swine; and 140 mg/kg for calves. Differences in LD_{50} values may be explained in part by the quality of the technical grade PCP used in the experiment.

Skin Absorption: The LD_{50} for rats has been reported as varying from 96 to 320 mg/kg and for mice as 261 mg/kg.

Inhalation: The LD_{50} by inhalation has been shown to be 225 mg/kg for rats and 355 mg/kg for mice. Human workers are known to have subjective complaints of the respiratory tract, particularly at very low concentrations of the chemical.

Clinical Effects: In animal exposures, experiments indicate that the animals will generally be found to have loss of appetite, diarrhea, stimulation of the central nervous system, increase in body temperature, acute renal failure, paralysis of the hind legs and changes in the cardiovascular system, any one of which might lead to death.

Chronic Studies

The "impure" commercial PCP has produced chloracne in rabbit ears and chick edema in bioassays. Studies of exposure of 90 days or more at dosages beginning at 10 mg/kg have been shown to cause increased liver weight and increased activity of microsomal liver enzymes, hepatocellular degeneration and necrosis, changes in liver enzymes, and decreases in hematological values. In one study, 25 ppm was considered to be the no effect level. Technical grade PCP containing significant amounts of dioxins and dibenzofurans has produced hepatic porphyria and increased hepatic aryl hydrocarbon hydroxylase activity, glucuronyl transferase activity, cytochrome P-450 and microsomal heme. Porphyria occurred at concentrations of 100 ppm. These changes were not all seen in the "pure" form of pentachlorophenol and were, therefore, felt to be the effects of the contaminating dioxins and dibenzofurans. Two year feeding studies have been performed with the report that at 25 to 30 mg/kg/day, the life span of the rats was not affected. However, at a dose of 30 mg/kg/day there were clear changes in both the liver and kidney which could be demonstrated.

Mutagenicity, Teratogenicity & Carcinogenicity Potential

Studies by Fahrig (1978) on pentachlorophenol containing impurities have not clearly demonstrated a mutagenic

effect. PCP has not shown mutagenic activity in the
Ames test, the host-mediated assay or the sex-linked
lethal test on drosophila. Further testing on chlorophenols will be required because of the possible mutagenic activity of the contaminants (Anderson, 1972;
Buselmeier, 1973; Vogel, 1974).

PCP has been found to be highly embryolethal at dosages of 16 mg/kg/day on days 6-15 of gestation in rats
with no effect produced at 5 mg/kg/day (Schwetz, 1974).
Oral Administration at 1.25 mg/kg/day in the days 5-10
of gestation in the golden Syrian hamster has caused
fetal deaths and PCP was found in the blood and fat of
fetuses (Hinkle, 1973). Technical grade PCP has been
implicated in causing teratogenic effects in women
(Kimbrough, 1972).

Rats maintained on diets of PCP for up to 24 months
did not develop cancer at diets sufficiently high to
cause mild signs of toxicity (1 mg/kg/day). Teratogenic
effects were not observed at dosages of 3 mg/kg/day although there was a decrease in neonatal survival and
growth among litters (Schwetz, 1978).

Human Illness Experience

Baader and Bauer (1951) reported ten cases of occupational illness in pentachlorophenol workers occurring in
a manufacturing plant in Germany. In addition to noting
the expected complaints of irritation of the mucous membranes of the respiratory tract, the cases were of interest in the report of peripheral neuritis and/or neuralgia,
tachycardia, dyspnea, elbow bursitis and loss of libido.
Interestingly, this report is the first to describe
chloracne in workers. In addition, the report notes that
the chloracne may have developed in half the workers
after the production process had ceased. The only other
report of occupationally related chloracne is that by
Nomura (1953).

Gordon (1956) reported a series of nine cases of pentachlorophenol intoxication. Five of these ended with
death, and only one was an episode of acute intoxication
following accidental ingestion. The remainder of the
cases are descriptions of a systemic illness from exposure in the field over a period of weeks with the gradual
onset of symptoms of recurrent abdominal pain, nausea,
vomiting, profuse sweating and elevated temperature.
These symptoms are now considered the typical complaints

associated with pentachlorophenol intoxication and are related in part to the ability of the chemical to un- couple oxidative phosphorylation. Autopsy studies in these cases revealed hepatic and renal congestion. In the case of inhalation, the author stated that there was also evidence of congestion and edema of the lungs.

Monon (1958) reported nine deaths as the result of chronic exposure to pentachlorophenol from workers dip- ping wood in a 1½-2% solution. Again, principal symptoms were hyperthermia, sweating, abdominal pain, shortness of breath and muscular spasm. Workers were exposed from three days minimum to 21 days maximum. No protective clothing or other simple hygienic measures were followed. An interesting sidelight to this report was that of the overseer on the job who, in order to convince the workers that the solution was not toxic, drank a glass of the 2% solution from the dispensing tank. He returned to work the following day complaining of a severe hangover, but was otherwise unaffected.

Several fatalities were also reported from South Africa by Blair (1961) and were related to a work team engaged in spraying water courses with PCP. Analyses for pentachlorophenol revealed levels of 5.9 to 6.2 mg/ 100 g of liver and 4.1 to 8.4 mg/100 g of kidney tissue. Levels in the blood ranged from 5.3 to 9.7 mg/100 ml and the level in the urine was reported as 2.8 mg/100 ml.

Other cases of pentachlorophenol intoxication have been reported such as that by Mason (1965) or by Bergner (1965). In all situations, most workers would agree that careful precautions should be taken in the occupational setting to prevent absorption via any route.

Measurement of Human Exposure

The Environmental Protection Agency currently has a program entitled, "The National Human Monitoring Program For Pesticides", whereby human urine is being analyzed for a variety of residues of selected pesticides and/or their metabolites. Preliminary analysis based upon 416 samples have demonstrated a mean of 6.3 ppb of penta- chlorophenol in about 85% of all samples tested with a maximum value of 193 ppb (Kutz, 1978).

In studies with occupationally exposed workers, Casarett and Bevenue (1969) have found levels ranging from 0.06 to 20.0 ppm. Studies by Wyllie (1975) perform- ed on workers in Idaho indicated levels in urine averaging 164 ppb for an exposed group and 3.4 ppb for a control group. Serum PCP levels ranged from 384.4 to 3,963 ppb for an exposed group and from 38.0 to 68.0 ppb for a control group. The average levels for the exposed and control groups were 1,372.1 ppb and 47.7 ppb respectively.

In cases of acute intoxication with PCP, a few studies have been reported giving levels found in human beings after fatality from an acute exposure. PCP in urine ranged from 28-96 ppm in post-mortem samples, according to a review by Bevenue and Beckman (1967a). Bevenue (1967b) also reported six cases of occupationally exposed pest control operators in Hawaii whose urinary PCP excretion exceeded 10 ppm without any findings of intoxication.

Armstrong (1969) reported an incident of PCP intoxication in St. Louis in which 20 infants developed symptoms secondary to PCP contamination of diapers. Nine cases of severe illness occurred, leading to fatality in two cases. Post-mortem tissue samples taken from one child contained 21-33 ppm of PCP. Serum levels of PCP in another infant ranged from 118 ppm prior to blood transfusion to 31 ppm on the following day. Serum levels of PCP in six exposed, but asymptomatic, infants ranged from 7-26 ppm. The concentration of PCP in the diapers used in the nursery ranged from 109-172 ppm.

First-Aid

Pentachlorophenol is usually absorbed through the skin when it is in the pure form. Absorption can probably also occur via the respiratory tract. In the event of body exposure, the skin should be thoroughly washed immediately. Wet clothing should be removed. If a spill occurs which involves the eyes, the chemical should be flushed out of the conjunctiva with copious amounts of water or saline.

In case of an accident in which the chemical has been swallowed, it is reasonable to induce vomiting but only if the patient is still alert and showing no signs of respiratory distress. A universal antidote, such as one which contains milk, cream or other materials of a fatty nature, should not be utilized since the lipophilic nature of the pentachlorophenol allows it to be absorbed into the antidote but also is then likely to be further absorbed in the gastrointestinal tract.

Diagnostic Studies

Urine is the appropriate tissue to be analyzed for pentachlorophenol levels. A few studies exist in the literature on serum, but these are not sufficient to establish any type of toxic level. Indeed, there is no level which can definitely be stated to be toxic in terms of urinary excretion. Fatal cases have shown 40-80 ppm of pentachlorophenol in the urine following acute exposure. On the other hand, the occupationally exposed individual may also excrete pentachlorophenol at levels of parts per million without complaints. Chemical blood studies should include careful assessment of both hepatic and renal involvement.

Specific Therapy and Follow-up

There is no specific antidote for pentachlorophenol intoxication. If PCP has been ingested, the stomach should be emptied. If the victim is still alert, Syrup of Ipecac may be utilized to induce vomiting. If the patient is not fully alert, the stomach should be intubated and aspiration should be performed using a saline or 5% sodium bicarbonate solution. Because the chemical is fat soluble and because the solvent is frequently a petroleum product, great care should be taken to prevent aspiration into the trachea. This should include the use of a cuffed endotrachial tube in the case of an unconscious patient. Following aspiration of the stomach contents, activated charcoal in water should be installed in the stomach as a means of limiting further absorption of PCP. Fat soluble cathartics should not be administered. If a cathartic is used, an osmotic type is preferable.

When the patient is hospitalized following the Emergency Room treatment, the patient should be observed carefully for evidence of hepatic, renal or central nervous system signs. Because of the hypermetabolic state induced, the body temperature will be elevated and attempts should be made to decrease it by sponge baths or cooling blankets. The use of antipyretics, such as aspirin, has been questioned and is considered to be contraindicated by some people with a preference to observe the febrile course as a means of monitoring the level of intoxication as well as the prevention of multiple drug interactions. Sedatives may be necessary to control central nervous system signs, particularly in the early stages, although

with severe intoxication, the patient can be expected to
gradually progress into a stuporous state. Both diaze-
pams and barbiturates have been used successfully although with the potential of the dioxin contaminants to
induce a porphyric state, the use of barbiturates seems
a rather questionable procedure. The gastrointestinal
complaints need to be handled purely on a symptomatic
basis via diet and antacids. Atropine is contraindicated
in the treatment of pentachlorophenol intoxication – as
opposed to the treatment of organophosphate intoxication
which may have rather similar presenting symptoms and
signs.

Occupational Hazards

    Although it would appear that the general public is
being exposed to pentachlorophenol either through food or
water, at this time there is no evidence that there is a
significant health problem associated with this type of
exposure. On the other hand, the worker who is daily
exposed to technical grade pentachlorophenol is at risk
for developing symptoms of chronic intoxication and pre-
cautionary measures are advised under these circumstances.
The chemical is highly irritating to the mucous membranes
and generally even small concentrations will be noxious
to employees. But, adaptation probably occurs with time
and therefore workers should be advised to wear respiratory protection. Safety glasses to prevent splashing
into the eyes are advisable. Clothing should be changed
regularly and spillage on clothing should be avoided
whenever possible. It should be recalled that the chemical in the pure form will easily absorb through the skin
and therefore protective gloves need to be utilized.
Contact dermatitis is possible in the worker who is repeatedly exposed to this chemical.

References

Ahling, B. and L. Johansson (1977) Combustion experiments using pentachlorophenol on a pilot scale and full-scale. Chemosphere 6:425.

Anderson, K.J. (1972) Evaluation of herbicides for possible mutagenic properties. J Agr Food Chem 20:649-656.

Armstrong, R.W., E.R. Eichner, D.E. Klein, W.F. Bartel, J.V. Bennett, V. Jonsson, H. Bruce and L.E. Loveless (1969) Pentachlorophenol poisoning in a nursery for newborn infants. II. Epidemiologic and toxicologic studies. J Pediatr 75:317-325.

Baader, E.W. and H.J. Bauer (1951) Industrial intoxication due to pentachlorophenol. Indust Med Surg 20:286-290.

Bergner, H. and P. Constantinidis (1965) Industrial pentachlorophenol poisoning in Winnipeg. Can Med Assoc J 92:448-451.

Bevenue, A. and H. Beckman (1967a) Pentachlorophenol: A discussion of its properties and its occurrences as a residue in human and animal tissues. Residue Rev 19:83-134.

Bevenue, A., T.J. Haley and H.W. Klemmer (1967b) A note on the effects of a temporary exposure of an individual to pentachlorophenol. Bull Environ Contam Toxicol 2:293-296.

Bevenue, A., J.R. Wilson, L.J. Casarett and H.W. Klemmer (1967c) A survey of pentachlorophenol content in human urine. Bull Environ Contam Toxicol 2:319-333.

Blair, D.M. (1961) Dangers in using and handling sodium pentachlorophenate as a molluscicide. Bull Wld Hlth Org 25:597-601.

Buselmeier, W. (1973) Comparative investigations on the mutagenicity of pesticides in mammalian test systems. Mutat Res 21:25-26.

Buser, H.R. (1976a) Higher resolution gas chromatography of polychlorinated dibenzo-p-dioxins and dibenzofurans. Anal Chem 48:1553.

Buser, H.R. and H.P. Bosshardt (1976b) Determination of polychlorinated dibenzo-p-dioxins and dibenzofurans in commercial pentachlorophenols by combined gas chromatography-mass spectrometry. J AOAC 59:562-569.

Casarett, L.J., A. Bevenue, W.L. Yauger, Jr. and S.A. Whalen (1969) Observations on pentachlorophenol in human blood and urine. Amer Ind Hyg Assoc J 30:360-366.

Crummett, W. and R.H. Stehl (1973) Determination of chlorinated dibenzo-p-dioxins and dibenzofurans in various materials. Environ Hlth Perspect 5:15.

Fahrig, R., C.A. Nilsson, C. Rappe (1978) Genetic activity of chlorophenols and chlorophenol impurities. IN: Pentachlorophenol, K.R. Rao (ed), Plenum Press, New York, pp. 325-328.

Gordon, D. (1956) How dangerous is pentachlorophenol? Med J Aust 2:485-488.

Hinkle, D.K. (1973) Fetotoxic effects of pentachlorophenol in the golden syrian hamster. Appl Pharmacol 25:455.

Kimbrough, R.D. (1972) Toxicity of chlorinated hydrocarbons and related compounds. Arch Environ Hlth 25:125-131.

Kutz, F.W., R.S. Murphy and S.C. Strassman (1978) Survey of pesticide residues and their metabolites in urine from the general population. IN: Pentachlorophenol, K.R. Rao (ed), Plenum Press, New York, pp. 363-369.

Mason, M.F. and S.M. Wallace (1965) Pentachlorophenol poisoning: Report of two cases. J Forensic Sci 10:136-147.

Menon, J.A. (1958) Tropical hazards associated with the use of pentachlorophenol. Br Med J 1:1156-1158.

Nilsson, C.A., A. Norstrom, K. Andersson and C. Rappe (1978) Impurities in commercial products related to pentachlorophenol. IN: Pentachlorophenol, K.R. Rao (ed), Plenum Press, New York, pp. 313-324.

Nomura, S. (1953) Studies on chlorophenol poisoning. J Sci Labour 29:474-483.

Schwetz, B.A., P.A. Keeler and P.J. Gehring (1974) The effect of purified and commercial grade pentachlorophenol on rat embryonal and fetal development. Toxicol Appl Pharmacol 28:151-161.

Schwetz, B.A. (1978) Results of two-year toxicity and reproduction studies on pentachlorophenol in rats. IN: Pentachlorophenol, K.R. Rao (ed), Plenum Press, New York, pp. 301-309.

Wyllie, J.A., J. Gabica, W.W. Benson and J. Yoder (1975) Exposure and contamination of the air and employees of a pentachlorophenol plant, Idaho - 1972. Pest Monit J 9:150-153.

2
Phenoxy Herbicides

Introduction

Among the most widely used of all herbicides are those chemicals which fall into the class of the chlorinated phenoxy compounds. These include particularly the herbicides 2,4,5-Trichlorophenoxyacetic acid (2,4,5-T) and 2,4-Dichlorophenoxyacetic acid (2,4-D). At the time of this writing, the use of the herbicide 2,4,5-T has been restricted by the Environmental Protection Agency and administrative hearings currently are underway raising numerous scientific issues regarding not only the use of 2,4,5-T, but many herbicides. There are important issues which have been raised by both the public and scientific community, such as the ability of some agricultural chemicals to be mutagenic, carcinogenic and teratogenic, in addition to their problems of acute toxicity. Furthermore, questions of hazard, risk and benefit are all part of issues which are currently being discussed.

In spite of 2,4,5-T presently being on a restricted list of chemicals, it is included in this section for several reasons. First of all, it is an agricultural chemical upon which many scientific studies have been performed and, therefore, it can be used to demonstrate the application of scientific data to the regulatory process. Secondly, some of the issues raised with 2,4,5-T will also be matters of importance with other agricultural chemicals, including 2,4-D.

2,4,5-Trichlorophenoxyacetic Acid

The chemical, 2,4,5-Trichlorophenoxyacetic acid,
commonly known as 2,4,5-T, has the structural formula
shown below.

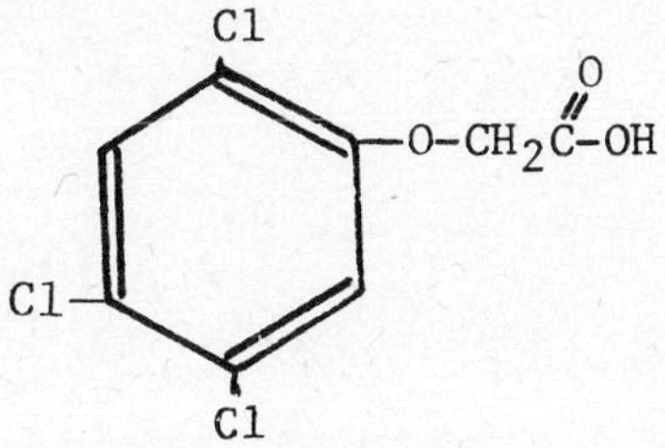

$$Cl$$

$$-O-CH_2\overset{\overset{O}{\|}}{C}-OH$$

$$Cl-$$

$$Cl$$

The pure acid is a white crystal and has a molecular
weight of 255.49. The melting point is 156.6°C. Its
solubility in water is 278 ppm at 25°C. It is also
soluble in acetone, ethanol, ether and alkaline solutions.
The esters of 2,4,5-T are emulsifiable in water and
soluble in most oils, while its amine salts are soluble
in water but insoluble in petroleum oils.
    The manufacturing process begins with 1,2,4,5-Tri-
chlorobenzene which is reacted with methanol and sodium
hydroxide to form 2,4,5-Trichlorophenol (2,4,5-TCP).
The TCP is then reacted with chloroacetic acid and with
sulfuric acid to produce 2,4,5-T. The acid form of
2,4,5-T can then be readily reacted with a variety of
alcohols to produce a number of esters or with amines to
produce amine salts.
    During the first step in the manufacturing process,
if temperatures are not carefully controlled, highly
toxic contaminants, the polychlorinated dibenzo-p-dioxins
can be formed. One of these, the tetrachlorodibenzo-p-
dioxin (TCDD) is the subject of widespread controversy
and will be dealt with in a separate section.

Registered Uses and Production

    The chemical 2,4,5-T is used as a selective herbicide,
especially for brush control. It can be used alone or is
commonly used mixed with other chemicals such as 2,4-D,
Dicamba, Picloram, Silvex, and MCPA. In 1970, approximately 12 million pounds were manufactured in the United
States but a considerable portion of this was exported.
The chemical is used principally on range land or
pasture and in forestry.

Metabolism in Experimental Animals

2,4,5-T may be excreted directly or degraded, with its primary degradation product occurring in the form of 2,4,5-Trichlorophenol. It has also been shown to be metabolized to derivatives of glycine and taurine. The degradation of 2,4,5-T in woody plants yields 2,4,5-TCP.

Environmental Fate

Regardless of route of application, 2,4,5-T remains principally upon the soil or foliage surface. It is easily bound by organic matter and, therefore, moves very poorly through most soils, although it will tend to move more in sandy soil. In the Pacific Northwest, a study by Norris (1969) showed that six months after the application of 2,4,5-T at two pounds per acre, the level of herbicide on the forest floor declined 90%. After one year, the level had declined more than 99%. The chemical remained in the upper 15 centimeters. Disappearance of the chemical probably occurred by volatilization as well as by bacterial degradation. When sprayed on soils, only small amounts are known to enter streams and again, studies by Norris (1967) in Oregon, have demonstrated that the maximum concentration after heavy spraying seldom exceeds 0.1 parts per million and this residue persisted for only a few hours. Upon entering streams, the chemical is probably lost by volatilization, degradation, absorption, biota and adsorption on bottom sediment. Because of its biodegradability, 2,4,5-T is not believed to bioaccumulate. A U.S. Geological Survey in 1965 studied a number of streams and was unable to detect 2,4,5-T with a lower limit of sensitivity at five parts per trillion. However, in studies of areas in which the water sheds have been sprayed with 2,4,5-T at four pounds per acre, levels of 2.1 parts per million were found one month after the spraying but within three months after application, there was no detectable level of 2,4,5-T.

Human Experiments

Gehring, et al (1973) have studied the absorption and excretion of 2,4,5-T following oral administration to five male volunteers at dosages of 5 mg/kg of analytical grade 2,4,5-T. These studies demonstrated that the

chemical follows a two compartment model with maximum
plasma concentrations being reached about seven hours
post-ingestion and reaching peak levels of about
60 mcg/ml (ppm). Excretion studies demonstrated first
order kinetics (exponential decay). At the end of 96
hours, 88.5±5.1% of the 2,4,5-T had been excreted unchanged in the urine. None of the five subjects became
ill following the experiment. Similar studies have also
been performed by Kohli (1974) from India in which human
volunteers were given dosages of 2, 3, or 5 mg/kg of
analytical grade 2,4,5-T. In this investigation, maximum
concentration reached approximately 25 mcg/ml at 7-24
hours after ingestion and then also declined in first
order kinetics. The half-life for plasma clearance was
estimated to be at 18.8±3.1 hours by Kohli and at 23.1
hours by Gehring. Somewhat similar studies have also
been performed by Matsumura (1970) with the ingestion of
100-150 mg of 2,4,5-T by human volunteers and again
demonstrating rapid absorption and elimination with more
than 80% of the original dose eliminated within 72 hours.

At the present time, The National Human Monitoring
Program For Pesticides is currently analyzing human urine
samples for Silvex, 2,4,5-T and 2,4,5-TCP. This survey
was scheduled for completion in 1979. To date, 400 urine
samples have been measured with no quantifiable 2,4,5-T
residues detected. Opposed to this is a study by
Dougherty (1976) at Florida State University who screened
the urine of students for chlorinated hydrocarbons and
felt that 2,4,5-T could be demonstrated in 9-36% of the
samples. This study has not yet been repeated and confirmed.

Incidental Human Exposure

The principal concern for human exposure is via the
food chain. Evidence that very little 2,4,5-T can get
into food has developed from results of the Market Basket Surveys conducted by the Food and Drug Administration. The first survey conducted from the years 1964
through 1969 with a total of 134 diet samples involving
1600 food composites demonstrated only three samples
which contained 2,4,5-T. Two of these were in dairy
products which contained a relatively high percentage of
fat, where the 2,4,5-T would be expected to accumulate.
The analyses demonstrated 0.008 and 0.19 ppm in the milk
fat. The remaining sample contained 0.003 ppm of

2,4,5-T on a fat basis in a meat, fish, and poultry composite.

The FDA Market Basket Survey performed in the years 1969 through 1974 showed no detectable 2,4,5-T residues (detection limit: 0.002 ppm) in 155 total diet samples involving 1,869 food composites. In the case of members of the public gardening on land adjacent to areas which have been sprayed with the chemical, there are no studies which have been performed to indicate the level of 2,4,5-T which might be present in that food although the level would be expected to be low - if present at all.

In areas adjacent to spraying operations, the water supply has also been demonstrated to contain the chemical for short periods of time immediately following the spraying as discussed earlier.

EPA's Pesticide Episode Response Branch has developed a system of collecting reports of pesticide exposure affecting humans, domestic animals, livestock and wildlife. According to their records, there were 98 episodes from 1966 to 1977 involving 2,4,5-T and 16 of these episodes concerned humans. Of these reported episodes, only two cases of human involvement could be documented and in both of these cases, 2,4-D was also involved. However, human illness, as opposed to exposure, has never been documented in the public at large. On the other hand, human illness is a concern to followers of human ecology and illness to synthetic agricultural chemicals in general has been alluded to in provocative testing methods by such authors as Randolph (1976) and Rea (1977).

Toxicology Studies

A summary of the scientific literature concerning 2,4,5-T has been published by Dost (1977) and the following is taken mainly from that source.

Acute toxicity: Studies in 1953 on dogs demonstrated an LD_{50} of about 100 mg/kg with the principal symptom being a mild incoordination. In male rats, the acute LD_{50} is 500 mg/kg; in male mice, 389 mg/kg; and in guinea pigs, 381 mg/kg. The LD_{50}'s for various esters are slightly higher than for the acid and the triethyl-amine salt of 2,4,5-T has been tested at 100 mg/kg with no observable effect.

Subacute and chronic toxicity studies: Subchronic
(90 day) feeding of male and female rats caused no effects below 30 mg/kg/day; body weight and food intake
were depressed with treatment at 100 mg/kg/day. At these
levels, alkaline phosphatase and SGPT were elevated and
erythrocytes and hemoglobin were decreased. In dogs fed
for five days weekly for a period of 90 days, dosages up
to 10 mg/kg/day were without effect but a dose of
20 mg/kg/day was lethal between 11 and 75 days after the
initiation of the experiment. In this case, symptoms
were limited to muscle twitching and impaired swallowing.
A two year feeding study of rats has shown that at dosages of 30 mg/kg/day the animals demonstrated an increased urinary porphyrin excretion after four months of
treatment and this change continued throughout the investigation. No other changes were found in hematological,
urinary tract or clinical chemistry parameters and increased porphyrin excretion did not occur at dosages of
10 or 3 mg/kg/day. Long-term studies on rodents have
been performed which demonstrate a variability in response between different strains. In the sensitive
strains of mice, myocardial lesions, bone marrow aplasia,
and lymphocytic depletion in the thymus, spleen and lymph
nodes were seen microscopically. These studies were
carried out at dosages of 60 mg/kg/day. With large doses,
2,4,5-T has also been found to increase liver weight in
rats and to impair secretion of itself by decreasing the
activity of the organic acid transport system at the
proximal tubule of the kidney. Based upon the above, the
conclusion is that the transport of phenoxy herbicides
through the kidney is an active process. Poultry seem
particularly insensitive to 2,4,5-T. Feeding a diet of
1,000 mg/kg/day to chicks showed only slight decrease in
growth rate but a 5,000 mg/kg diet was lethal. Turkeys
fed 2,4,5-T at 62 mg/day were unaffected.
The material below on acute toxicity has been summarized by the Forest Service - USDA (1977).

Acute Toxicity of 2,4,5-T

Organism	2,4,5-T
Birds:	
LD_{50}	300
No effect, ppm	600
Rodents:	
LD_{50}, mg/kg	400–950
No effect, ppm	800
Ruminants:	
LD_{50}, mg/kg	500–1,000
No effect, ppm	1,200
Other mammals:	
LD_{50}, mg/kg	100
No effect, ppm	200
Fish:	
TL_m, ppm	1–30
No effect, ppm	0.1
Other aquatics:	
TL_m, ppm	0.5–50
No effect, ppm	0.05

Teratogenicity

The teratogenic potential of 2,4,5-T, and of its contaminant tetrachlorodibenzo-p-dioxin (TCDD), is clearly
one of the most volatile and widely discussed issues
relating to the use of this herbicide. A review of the
literature on teratogenicity of 2,4,5-T is complicated
not only by the fact that TCDD is present in the commercial product but also because the percentage of TCDD has
been markedly reduced since the chemical was first used
as an herbicide. Initially, 2,4,5-T contained up to
30 ppm of TCDD contaminant and initial studies of potential teratogenicity of 2,4,5-T were, therefore, based
upon dose-response curves with material containing the
two chemicals in significant quantity. Present manufacturing methods have decreased the amount of TCDD to a
level of 0.02 ppm in the 2,4,5-T formulation, although
the law allows for a maximum of 0.1 ppm. Initially, the

use of this chemical in Viet Nam as a defoliant led to concern that fetal malformations might be occurring in the Vietnamese population. This concern was allayed, to some degree, as the result of a special study team of the National Academy of Sciences which reported no changes in congenital malformations, but this report has been criticized and not totally accepted. The principal reason behind such criticism probably lies in the difficulty of the study team to procur good records from an underdeveloped country in the midst of a full-scale war. The records studied were from the hospital population in Saigon, whereas, the defoliated zone was about 50 miles away.

In experimental studies with commercial 2,4,5-T of present-day quality, the no observable effect level for teratogenesis in rats is considered to be 20 mg/kg/day with feeding studies that proceed through the significant early days of gestation. Studies with dosages of 24, 40, and 50 mg/kg/day have not demonstrated teratogenicity. In mice, the teratogenic dose is similar to that of rats with dosages at 50 mg/kg/day showing evidence of increased frequency of cleft palates as well as resorption frequency of the fetus. Hamsters, rabbits, and ruminants are more resistant to teratogenic effects. Dougherty (1975) administered 0.5, 1.0, and 10 mg/kg/day to groups of 10 pregnant rhesus monkeys and teratogenic effects were not demonstrated. Studies on eggs indicate that the possibility of eggs developing a teratogenic dose of 2,4,5-T seems highly unlikely. On the other hand, non-mammalian species may be more sensitive to 2,4,5-T. In one study on insects, a disturbed egg follicle development and chromosomal defect in a diet containing 1 ppm was shown. Similarly, a study in fish has demonstrated that concentrations of 20 ppm may have a substantial teratogenic effect.

Concern for human exposure arises from the possibility of exposure and significant absorption of the chemical – unless one assumes that any amount of chemical, no matter how small, is a significant health hazard. The principal route of exposure must come from skin absorption and could only occur in situations where humans are sprayed directly, either in working conditions or accidentally. At the present time, the safety of aerial application is the most widely debated issue. The Working Group which directed that 2,4,5-T would be placed on the RPAR list addressed this issue and published their findings in the Federal Register of April 21, 1978. Their calculations were based upon the hypothetical situation that a spray plane would fly directly over a person who would have bare skin of the head, neck, shoulders, forearms, hands and thighs. If the person were thoroughly saturated and an assumed absorption of 10% of the material occurred, an estimated dose level would be 0.051 mg/kg in a 60 kg woman. This compares with the no adverse effect level for teratogenic effects of 20 mg/kg. The conclusion of the Working Group was that the calculated dermal exposure did not constitute an ample margin of safety. (200 times less than the calculated no effect level.) The assumptions were admittedly worst possible case and in their calculations an application made of four pounds of acid equivalent 2,4,5-T per acre was used. In industrial practices, such as forestry, the actual dosage used is usually one to two pounds per acre of acid equivalent 2,4,5-T. The calculated dermal exposures from this follow – with corrections made to bring the dosage from exposure to one pound per acre – and are compared against calculated exposures to TCDD under the identical circumstances.

Dermal Exposure (Aerial Application)

	2,4,5-T	TCDD
Use dilution rate	1 lb 2,4,5-T/ 10 gallons of water/acre	0.0000001 lb TCDD/ 10 gallons of water/acre
% diluted material absorbed	10%	10%
Exposure level	0.8 mg	0.00008 ug
Dose level	0.013 mg/kg	1×10^{-6} ug/kg
No adverse effect level for teratogenic effects	20 mg/kg	0.03 ug/kg

Although oral and inhalation exposures are nowhere near as potentially dangerous or as significant as dermal exposure, figures have been calculated to determine what amount of food, contaminated with the maximum allowable concentration of 2,4,5-T, would need to be ingested. The following table from the Yarram, Australia Report (1978)

reflects the amount of food which would be required per
day during the susceptible part of the gestational
period in order to reach the no adverse effect level for
teratogenesis in the most susceptible animal. Note that
in each case (oral or dermal), the toxicity of 2,4,5-T is
more important than that of TCDD. This is because of the
relatively low concentration of TCDD in the parent compound as compared against the toxicities in experimental
animals of the two chemicals.

Source	2,4,5-T		TCDD	
Spray mix	1.5	1	22.5	1
Blackberries	24	kg	360	kg
Water	60,000	1	900,000	1
Milk	12,000	1	180,000	1
Meat	6,000	kg	90,000	kg

A recent article by Nelson and coworkers (1979) was
directed at the occurrence of cleft palate in Arkansas
and a possible relationship to the agricultural use of
2,4,5-T. Estimated levels of exposure to 2,4,5-T were
determined by categorizing 75 Arkansas counties into
high, medium, or low exposure groups and a total of
1,201 cases of cleft lip and/or cleft palate were reviewed. Facial cleft rates, presented by sex, race, time and
exposure group, generally rose over a period of time but
no significant differences were found for any race or sex
combination and the gradual increase in cleft palate incidence could not be attributed to maternal exposure to
2,4,5-T. The study does not resolve the question of
cause and effect between 2,4,5-T and cleft palate since
a two-fold increase would have been needed to detect a
change and the authors believe that a final conclusion
could only be reached if 2,4,5-T epidemiological studies
could be performed with very accurate assessment of
exposure.

Carcinogenic and Mutagenic Potential of 2,4,5-T

Because of the ever present contaminating dioxin,
TCDD, in formulations of 2,4,5-T, the studies on the
carcinogenic or mutagenic potential of 2,4,5-T cannot be
singly evaluated.

In experimental animals, 2,4,5-T has not been shown to
have carcinogenic potential. In a study involving the
screening of 120 pesticides and industrial chemicals published by Innes, et al (1969), none of the phenoxy herbicides, including 2,4,5-T, caused increased tumor formation after a maximum tolerable daily dose over 20 days.
Muranyi-Kovacs, et al (1976) treated mice with 80 ppm
2,4,5-T for more than 500 days at a daily dosage of
12-15 mg/kg. In one strain, survival time was significantly decreased in the males and in another strain,
significantly increased in the females. In those animals
that had an increased life span, there appeared to be a
small increase in tumor incidence but the conclusion is
that the altered life span confounded the analysis and,
therefore, that 2,4,5-T (including the TCDD contaminant
at 0.05 ppm) required further study.

In human beings, the most frequently cited study on
phenoxy acid exposure (2,4-D and 2,4,5-T) is that by
Axelson and Sundell (1974). This was a study on Swedish
railroad workers with exposure to a variety of herbicides
with results that are still open to question. These
workers appeared to demonstrate a significantly increased
tumor incidence and tumor mortality. The excess of
tumors was found particularly among workers with exposure
to amitrol (aminotriazole) with the original conclusion
reached that the amitrol exposure may have caused the
excess of tumors. A re-analysis by the Work Group of the
IARC (1978) suggests that the phenoxy acids "show a possible and previously masked tumor-inducing effect". Furthermore, in an update of the Swedish railroad workers
published by Axelson (1979), an excess of tumors of the
stomach in the phenoxy acid exposed workers was found
(2 observed versus 0.33 expected). In "herbicide exposed
workers" a variety of other herbicide exposures also
occurred during the period of 1957-1961, but there was a
significant excess total mortality (31 observed versus 22
expected) and also a significant excess of all tumors (14
observed versus 5.44 expected).

A follow-up by Hardell and Sandstrom (1979) on patients
admitted to the Department of Oncology at the University
Hospital in Umea, Sweden during the years 1970-1977 demonstrated an increased relative risk and the development
of malignant mesenchymal tumors among men occupationally
exposed to phenoxyacetic acid. In addition, a study by
Hardell (1980) of patients admitted during the years
1974-1978 showed an increased risk for the development of
Hodgkin's disease or non-Hodgkin's lymphoma in men

exposed to phenoxy acids.

By contrast, a retrospective cohort mortality study conducted in Finland on workers involved in spraying 2,4-D and 2,4,5-T did not show any increase in mortality during the period of 1955-1971. A prospective follow-up study for the period 1972-1976 revealed fewer cancer-related deaths than expected in all age groups. However, clinical and anamestic investigations performed during this study did show a picture of an acute clinical syndrome during and following spraying operations consisting of: headache, transient dizziness, fatigue, abdominal complaints, skin and mucous irritations and a few cases of persistent papulae (IARC, 1978).

Finally, a study by Ott, et al (1980) on employees engaged in the manufacture of 2,4,5-T demonstrated no excess in overall mortality and a lower than expected death rate due to malignant neoplasm. The study by Ott is the only one where attempts were made to quantify exposure rather than simply assess whether exposure had indeed occurred.

It seems reasonable to conclude that the situation regarding occupational exposure to the phenoxy herbicides and any association with cancer is still not clear. The Swedish studies have been criticized for a lack of quantification and specificity, nevertheless, the finding of a rare type of tumor in these workers does appear documented. On the other hand, studies in Finland, as well as by Ott, would indicate that no statistical association can be observed between occupational exposure to the phenoxy herbicides and increased risk for cancer.

Hardell (1977) reported results from Sweden on a study of patients suffering from mesenchymal tumors without occupational or other exposures to phenoxy acid. During the years 1970 through 1976, 87 mesenchymal tumors were diagnosed. Of these cases, 55 were men and 43 of these 55 men were known by profession: 19 were either forestry workers, farmers and forestry workers, or workers in sod mills and paper mills where exposure to chlorophenols is common. Based upon the official statistics of Sweden, and calculating the approximate expected fraction of tumors within these grades, the expectancy for these tumors would have been approximately 11 cases as versus the 19 observed.

In experimental systems, 2,4,5-T has not been shown to be a mutagen. The compound has not induced mutants in a variety of bacterial systems. In Drosophila, 2,4,5-T did show increased sex linked recessive lethal mutations

after 15 day feedings. Up to 150 mg/kg of 2,4,5-T
produced no increase in chromosomal abnormalities
although higher doses did cause some increase.

In human beings, a survey of pesticide applicators who
had been in contact with a wide variety of agents was
published by Yoder, et al (1975) and appeared to show
some increase in chromatid gaps and breaks during the
spray season. This was followed by recovery in the off-
season with a reduced frequency below that of a control
time, suggesting some type of repair system. In this
study, 2,4,5-T was not a frequently used agent among the
many that the workers were exposed to and the effect
could not be specifically attributed to that chemical
alone. These studies have not been repeated on other
workers. The Dow Chemical Company has maintained a program of monitoring on 2,4,5-T production workers and
cytogenetic evaluations of 52 men in early 1970 were reported to be negative by Johnson (1971). A second analysis by Kilian (1974) was also found to be negative.

Symptoms and Signs of Injury or Intoxication

Years of experience with 2,4,5-T have led most occupational physicians to believe that this compound is relatively innocous to human beings although absorption can
occur by all three routes. Skin exposure can lead to
primary skin irritation and also to allergic contact
dermatitis. Protracted inhalation of the spray will act
as a primary irritant of the mucous membranes of the respiratory tract leading to secondary complaints of burning
sensations, cough, lacrimation and rhinitis. Inhalation
has also been related to complaints of dizziness and
ataxia of a transient nature, however, these complaints
may be related to aromatic hydrocarbons which are used as
a solvent. It is believed that if this compound were ingested, irritation of the mouth and throat would occur
and probably gastrointestinal irritation would follow
which would lead to nausea, vomiting and chest pain
secondary to esophagitis (not cardiac in origin). If
intestinal irritation were severe enough, abdominal pain,
tenderness and diarrhea could ensue.

In fact, there have been no documented cases of systemic intoxication ever reported in the medical literature
with the use of 2,4,5-T. Therefore, suspected symptoms
of intoxication are based principally upon experimental
studies in animals rather than clinical experience. Based

upon these types of studies, one might also expect the
possibility of increased muscle tone and fibrillations
as a principal manifestation of most systemic intoxication.

In industrial workers, a symptom complex principally
manifested as a development of chloracne but also with
the possibilities of developing porphyria cutanea tarda,
hepatic injury, gastrointestinal complaints and peripheral neuropathy has been shown to occur. This symptom
complex may be related to the contaminant TCDD and is
discussed in more detail in the section on dioxin.

Diagnostic Studies

Under normal circumstances, human beings should not
have any evidence of 2,4,5-T present either in their
urine or in their plasma. Lavy (1978) reported an investigation of 2,4,5-T applicators. Absorption of
2,4,5-T was estimated on the basis of urinary excretion.
The workers excreted 0.002 mg/kg to 0.07 mg/kg, depending
upon their occupation, i.e. the mixers and backpack
sprayers clearly had the most absorption. The analyses
can be performed without difficulty using gas chromatography. Either urine (minimum of 300 cc's - 24 hour
sample preferred) or plasma (minimum of 10 cc's) should
be used for the analysis. Following an acute exposure,
it should be remembered that the compound has a rapid
phase of excretion which occurs within the first 24 to 48
hours and then is followed by a continued, but much lower, rate of excretion until no observable levels are seen.

Because of the possibility of co-existing dioxin
contamination, studies should be performed on hepatic
function, urinary excretion of porphyrin and studies
demonstrating heart and neurological deficits, e.g. EMG.

First Aid

1. Remove patient from contact and remove contaminated clothing. If symptoms of illness
   occur following inhalation of spray, the
   individual should not be allowed subsequent
   use of chlorophenoxy compounds unless effective respiratory protection is also utilized.

2. Bathe and shampoo with soap and water to remove chemicals and prevent further absorption.
   Individuals who have chronic skin disease
   should not be allowed to work with this chemical because of increased probability of
   dermal absorption.

3. In case of spillage into the eyes, clean
   water or isotonic saline should be used to
   flush the eyes for 10-15 minutes.

4. If ingested, and if the patient is fully
   alert, emesis should be induced.

Specific Therapy

It must be re-emphasized that since acute intoxication
has not occurred in human beings, the following recommendations for specific treatment are conjectural and based
upon best assumptions.

1. If patient is alert, emesis should be induced
   using an agent such as Syrup of Ipecac. If
   the level of consciousness is decreased, the
   possibility of respiratory inhalation must be
   considered. The latter may be particularly
   dangerous because of the presence of petroleum
   distillates which are commonly used as solvents.
   In this case, the stomach should be emptied by
   intubation, aspiration and lavage.

2. After induced emesis or aspiration of the
   stomach, washing with isotonic saline or
   sodium bicarbonate is recommended. Following this, the administration of activated
   charcoal in water would be useful. It should
   be remembered that in cases of intoxication
   the stomach contents should be kept for
   future analysis.

3. Administer saline cathartic.

4. If absorption with secondary symptoms are
   believed to have occurred, it has been recommended that glucose in an electrolyte solution be administered intravenously to

accelerate excretion. Theoretically, frank
alkanization may be appropriate (see treatment of 2,4-D). Although the compound is
believed to be excreted via the renal tubules,
the role of such agents as Mannitol or other
commonly used diuretics, such as ethacrynic
acid, thiazides, etc., is not known.

5. Observe the patient for evidence of injury
   to the kidneys, liver, gastrointestinal
   tract, central and peripheral nervous system.
   Treat patient with supportive measures and
   for symptomatic relief of complaints.

2,4-Dichlorophenoxyacetic Acid

The Chemical and Physical Characteristics

The chemical, 2,4-Dichlorophenoxyacetic acid, commonly
known as 2,4-D, has the structural formula shown below.

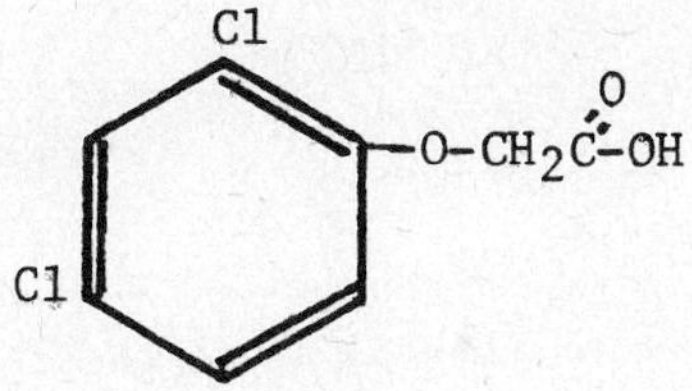

The empirical formula is $C_8H_6Cl_2O_3$. The molecular weight
is 221.04. The chemical is a crystalline, colorless and
odorless (when pure) compound. The melting point is
141°C and the boiling point is 160°C at 0.4 mm Hg. The
pure chemical is soluble in water at 540 ppm at 20°C,
soluble in alkali, highly soluble in benzene, carbon
tetrachloride and other organic solvents. The chemical
is stable in solutions as well as in the crystalline
state although slight decomposition will occur with
ultraviolet irradiation. Solubility will vary considerably depending upon the nature of the manufactured salt.
Presently, the preferred process of manufacture is the
gradual chlorination of phenol. This leads to a product
which is predominantly 2,4-dichlorophenol at temperatures
slightly above 43°C. Under usual manufacturing conditions

a product which is 92-98% pure may be obtained, with the major contaminants being 2,6-dichlorophenol and 0.5% 2,4,6-trichlorophenol. However, in the second step of manufacture, known as the condensation step, monochloro-acetic acid is reacted with the 2,4-dichlorophenol to achieve the end product. This condensation step is carried out under alkaline conditions and the waste products of manufacture from 2,4-D have been shown to contain 2,7-dichlorodibenzo-p-dioxin at concentrations of approximately 300 ppm (Goulding et al, 1972). The purity of technical 2,4-D was examined by Woolson (1972). With 28 samples of 2,4-D, only one sample gave a positive finding for any dioxin and this represented a response for hexa-chlorodioxin at a level of less than 10 ppm. Studies by Cochrane (1980) have demonstrated that commercial 2,4-D contains not only the expected 2,7-dichlorodibenzo-p-dioxin, but also contains lesser amounts of both a tri-chloro- and a tetrachloro-dioxin. Importantly, the 2,3,7,8-TCDD is not a contaminant of 2,4-D.

Registered Uses and Production

2,4-D is registered both as an herbicide for the control of broadleaf plants and as a plant growth regulator. A number of fruit and vegetable crops are registered for its use and in the Pacific Northwest, wheat production is one of the major applications. Non-crop use includes: application to aquatic sites, fallow land, lawns and turfs, reforestation projects, ditch banks, potential range lands, rights of way, fence rows or similar sites. As a growth regulator, 2,4-D is used on citrus crops to increase fruit size, reduce drop and delay ripening or degreening. It is used on lemons to delay fungus infestation in storage. It is also used to improve the skin appearance of potatoes by intensifying the red color.

In 1973, approximately 40-50 million pounds of 2,4-D were used domestically. Approximately two-thirds was used in agriculture and the remaining was used for non-agricultural uses.

Environmental Fate

2,4-D is not persistent in soil or water and is believed to break down within four to six weeks after application in soil. A national soils monitoring program which covered crop land in 43 states and non-crop land in 11 states was summarized by Wiersma (1972). Of 188 samples analyzed, only three were found to be positive, with a range of 0.01-0.03 ppm, and these data suggest that 2,4-D is relatively non-persistent in most soil types.

In water, the half-life of 2,4-D is believed to be about six days. Contamination of aquatic sites due to surface runoff or soil erosion is believed to be unlikely, both because of the short half-life of 2,4-D in soil and because the chemical does not move well through soil. Nevertheless, aquatic contamination can occur via aerial drift or from direct application to water for weed control. Studies performed on water samples in areas where 2,4-D was applied terrestrially have shown levels as high as 100 ppb shortly following application although the usual levels are even less than this. Lake mud microbial action and ultraviolet light decompose 2,4-D. Thus, 2,4-D is believed to be present only in trace amounts after one month.

Movement of 2,4-D in air does occur and it may drift via air currents for considerable distances from the application site. This may be the direct result of the air application or it may be the result of volatilization from the target area.

Metabolism in Experimental Animals

2,4-D can be expected to be rapidly absorbed from both the lungs and the gastrointestinal tract. Studies in rabbits by Kay (1965) would indicate that 2,4-D is only poorly absorbed through the skin. The chemical is believed to be excreted rapidly from the body and the half-life is in the range of four to six hours. By 30-48 hours, the chemical is barely, if at all, found at detectable levels in tissues of animals with the 2,4-D excreted almost entirely unchanged through the urine.

Animal Toxicology Studies

Acute: Hill and Carlisle (1947) have established LD_{50} values for a variety of animal species: mice, 375 mg/kg; rats, 666 mg/kg; rabbits, 800 mg/kg; guinea pigs, 1000 mg/kg. In non-lethal doses, the animals develop a neurological sign such as gross incoordination

and myotonia. Other manifestations include diarrhea and
respiratory irritation. The report by Hill and Carlisle
cites that monkeys were able to tolerate 214 mg/kg without severe residual effect, however, twice that dose
caused expected symptoms of vomiting and incoordination.
Strangely enough, a loss of muscle tone, rather than increased muscular tone, occurred. In dogs, observations
by Drill and Hiratzka (1953) have set an LD_{50} at 100 mg/
kg.

Chronic: Hansen, et al (1971) studied the chronic
toxicity of 2,4-D in both rats and dogs. Starting at
three weeks of age, rats were fed up to 1,250 ppm of
2,4-D for two years with no significant effect on growth
rate, survival rate, organ weights or hematologic values.
No carcinogenic effect occurred. Beagle dogs were fed up
to 500 ppm of 2,4-D in the diet starting at 6-8 months of
age. No 2,4-D related effects were noted. Finally, a
three-generation six-litter reproduction study was carried out with dietary 2,4-D at 100 to 500 ppm with no
deleterious effects seen. At 1,500 ppm, however, 2,4-D
reduced the percent of pups born surviving to weaning
and reduced the weight of weanlings.
    A variety of long-term studies have been performed
using grazing animals and domesticated wildlife. These
studies have been summarized by Dost (1977). Daily oral
dosages of 10 mg/kg to 100 mg/kg are required to produce
significant signs of toxicity in cattle, sheep and chickens.

Teratogenicity

    The first published study on teratogenic responses in
rats was published by Schwetz, et al (1971). Pregnant
rats were treated with 2,4-D at dosage levels of 12.5-
87.5 mg/kg/day (maximum tolerated dose). Foetotoxic
effects were seen at higher dosages and the author suggested that the dose level without effect would be
25 mg/kg/day for 2,4-D.
    Studies by Khera (1972) show foetotoxic and teratogen-
ic effects, particularly with the ester derivatives of
2,4-D. The low dose required to produce these effects is
estimated at 100 mg/kg with a no observable effect level
at 50 mg/kg. Collins, et al (1971) studied pregnant hamsters and fed doses of 2,4-D ranging from 0-100 mg/kg on
day 6-10 of gestation. Terata were occasionally produced

and the lowest dose causing fetal anomalies was 60 mg/kg or approximately 600 ppm in the diet.

Because of concern that eggs might be particularly susceptible, Grolleau, et al (1974) studied the effect of application of 2,4-D by spraying on quail eggs at three different dosages, the lowest dose corresponding to normal environmental levels after foliage treatment. No detrimental effect was seen. Experimentation with partridge included histopathological examination of the tissue but, again, no discernible effects were noted. Bage, et al (1973) in studies in Sweden concluded that 2,4-D is teratogenic at high dosages of above 110 mg/kg/day. In reviewing previous data, these investigators feel that the dose resulting in teratogenic effects from 2,4-D is extremely high as compared with the dose to which a pregnant woman could normally be exposed. Thus, the results of their studies seem to indicate to them that no special risk to the human embryo from the regular use of phenoxy herbicides exists.

Carcinogenicity and Mutagenicity of 2,4-D

The study by Hansen, et al (1971) was carried out over a period of two years without evidence of 2,4-D being carcinogenic. In addition, there is a screening study by Innes, et al (1969) in which 2,4-D and several of its esters were also not shown to be carcinogenic. A carcinogenic potential via in vitro experiments has been demonstrated by Seiler (1979) and Walker, et al (1972) whereby it would appear that 2,4-D has the ability to inhibit DNA synthesis. For more discussion see the 2,4,5-T-carcinogen section.

2,4-D has not been demonstrated to be mutagenic. The Ames test, performed by Anderson, et al (1972), did not detect mutagenic activity. Jenssen and Renberg (1976) found that 2,4-D had no effect upon cytogenetic tests as judged by increase in micronuclei erythrocytes. They concluded that their experiment demonstrated lack of cytogenetic hazard in man. Studies by Zetterberg, et al (1977) on genetic effect of 2,4-D in yeast cells and bacteria were negative and no genetic effects were induced by oral administration of 2,4-D in host-mediated assays using mice as host and yeast or Salmonella as indicator·cells.

Human Toxicology

The pharmacokinetics of 2,4-D in man have been studied by Sauerhoff and co-workers (1977). Five subjects ingested a single dose of 5 mg/kg 2,4-D without any detectable clinical effects. Excretion occurred via the urinary tract with an average half-life of 18 hours. The excretion of 2,4-D from plasma occurred with an average half-life of 12 hours. After ingestion, plasma concentrations reached a peak of approximately 25 mcg/ml (ppm) after four hours.

Based upon the above investigation, the authors conclude that repeated administration of the chemical would lead to a steady-state concentration of 2,4-D in approximately three days, i.e. seven times the biological half-life. Following this time, no additional accumulation would occur in spite of the continued ingestion at the same dose rate.

As with 2,4,5-T, there are no documented cases of intoxication from 2,4-D in the public occurring as the result of incidental exposure. However, unlike 2,4,5-T, there are a number of cases of intoxication resulting from 2,4-D which have either occurred with the use of the chemical or as the result of accidental ingestion or suicidal attempts.

Industrially, one of the most frequently cited studies are the consecutive studies of industrially acquired porphyria reported initially by Bleiberg (1971) with a follow-up article by Poland (1971). These studies have been commented upon in the section on dioxin since the porphyria and majority of other symptoms are now believed to be secondary to the dioxins rather than the phenoxy-acetic acids.

The first suggestion that occupational use of 2,4-D after several weeks of application might lead to a clinical illness was briefly reported in the Correspondence section of JAMA in 1956. Then, Goldstein, et al (1959) reported three cases of severe sensory and motor symptoms occurring in two men and one woman following what appeared to be only incidental exposure, i.e. 10 cc's of spill on the forearms without washing. In addition to the involvement of the peripheral nervous system, there seemed to be some symptoms and signs of a rather generalized toxic reaction manifested principally as headache, nausea and vomiting, vertigo and fatigue. These cases were not immediately accepted because the question arose as to whether the syndrome was really secondary to the petroleum vehicle used with 2,4-D or was a result of the chemical itself. Todd (1962) reported the case of a 52 year old male who also developed an illness which was gastrointestinal with nausea, vomiting and diarrhea lasting for approximately ten days, and, which was also neurological. The latter syndrome was consistent with peripheral neuropathy involving the upper and lower extremities, loss of proprioception, loss of deep tendon reflexes, muscular paralysis or paresis and the absence of pathological reflexes. The syndrome lasted for approximately two years. Berkley and Magee (1963) reported the case of a 39 year old farmer who used an automatic sprayer on his tractor and exposed himself to 2,4-D without making any attempt to wash the chemical off. Four days after this exposure, he developed symptoms of numbness and tingling of the hands and toes, generalized weakness with development of moderate incoordination, decreased position and vibratory sensation and loss of deep tendon reflexes. Although they gradually improved, symptoms persisted for no less than eight months.

Nielsen, et al (1965) reported the first case of death secondary to 2,4-D suicide. An estimated six grams of 2,4-D was ingested, corresponding to a dose of about 80 mg/kg. Tissue analysis showed relatively high levels of 2,4-D in the blood, liver and intestine. Very low levels were found in the central nervous system. In terms of absolute measurements, large amounts of 2,4-D were found in the muscle, liver and blood. In spite of the relatively low central nervous system levels, distinct changes in both gross and microscopic pathology were seen in the brain, principally as paravascular hemorrhages and pericellular edema and as severe degenerative changes of the ganglion cells. Levels of 2,4-D expressed as mg/g of organ weight varied from a low of 12.5 in the brain to 183 in the liver, 669 in the blood and 270 in the urine.

Geldmacher-v. Mallinckrodt and Lautenbach (1966) reported two successful suicidal attempts from a mixture of 2,4-D and MCPA. Symptoms were principally of the central nervous system with one patient eventually dying from a secondary pneumonitis and the second dying with hyperthermia. Dosages could not be determined. Concentrations in the blood varied from 2.3-4.2 mg% which indicated a very high intake.

An instructive case of suicide in a retired forestry professor who ingested approximately one pint of what is believed to be "pure" 2,4-D dissolved in an unknown quantity of kerosene is described by Dudley and Thapar (1972). The clinical triad of gastroenteritis, skeletal and cardiac myotonia, and central nervous system depression followed the experience of previous reports. Tissue concentrations in various organs were: blood, 57 ppm; brain, 93 ppm; kidney, 193 ppm; liver, 407 ppm; and muscles 117 ppm. At autopsy, the authors noted evidence of acute demyelination in all parts of the brain.

Another interesting report of 2,4-D intoxication is that by Berwick (1970) who reported an illness following the accidental ingestion of 30 ml of the concentrated chemical. Again, the triad of gastrointestinal, muscular and central nervous system complaints developed. Of interest in this case was the documentation of rhabdomyolisis with striking elevations in muscular enzymes, not only CPK and aldolase but also LDH, SGOT and SGPT. In addition, the urine was found to have levels of oxymyoglobin and oxyhemoglobin. In this case, the patient made a complete recovery and 36 months later, he had no signs or symptoms of either central or peripheral nervous system disease. During the course of the acute illness, respiratory problems developed as the result of paralysis of the intercostal muscles. A report by Davies and Jung (1976) in which 40 ml of a commercial herbicide was ingested prosents a less severe picture. However, in the latter report, the clinical picture is complicated by a pneumonitis which may be the result of either aspiration following haematemisis and/or poor respiratory excursions as the result of the involvement of the skeletal muscles.

In spite of the above case reports, it would appear, both from occupational experience and the experience in the general public, that the risk of intoxication syndromes with 2,4-D is of a low incidence. Of particular interest is the report by Seabury (1963) of two cases of terminally ill patients with coccidiomycosis who were given the sodium salt of 2,4-D as a form of treatment. One of these patients received the dose intramuscularly and only received a total of 40 mg prior to death. The second case, however, received the drug intravenously, the most dangerous route of all and one which would be expected to give signs very quickly. This patient received 2,4-D intravenously daily in increasing amounts until a dose of 2,000 mg in two hours was reached with no obvious reaction. When a dose of 3,600 mg was given intravenously, the patient experienced fibrillary twitchings of the mouth and upper extremities, plus generalized hyporeflexia. By this time, the patient had received a

total dose of 12.7 grams. Following the dosage of 3,600
mg, no further 2,4-D was administered and the patient
lived another 17 days with findings of marked muscular
weakness and lethargy. The latter findings may not have
been related to the use of 2,4-D since the patient was
pre-terminally ill from his primary disease. At autopsy,
the only findings were those of generalized coccidiomycosis and secondary tissue changes ascribed to that disease.

First Aid

In the case of a spill with secondary dermal contact,
the skin should be immediately washed with soap and water
or well flushed. Any chemical in the mucous membrane
should be flushed out, particularly in the eyes. In the
case of ingestion, it is reasonable to force emesis if
the patient is awake. Again, if the vehicle is a petroleum solvent, the dangers of inhalation pneumonitis must
be considered.

Diagnostic Studies

Normally, body tissues do not contain a level of 2,4-D.
In the case of exposure, either occupational or otherwise,
measurement in the urine would appear to be the simplest
procedure; although whole blood can also be utilized. In
occupational workers, the safety factor is large and, in
most cases, workers will not excrete 2,4-D even after a
working day. Batchmen (mixers) are particularly liable
to have absorption, as are pilots. Minimal safety factors
for crewmen such as long sleeve shirts, hats and boots
seem to be more than ample to protect workers from any
absorption and the safety factor, even with the unprotected worker, is better than 1,000:1. Exposure levels
performed by Lavy (1980) indicate an estimated average
dose of 2,4-D ranging from 0.0049 to 0.0198 mg/kg/24
hours in the unprotected worker. In most occupational
workers, one should not expect a level to exceed 1.0 ppm
in a random urine. There are no established levels above
which one can state that toxicity is likely to be present.
In the case of intoxication syndromes, serial bloods or
urines should be collected and used to monitor treatment.
As in the case with 2,4,5-T, there is a rapid phase of
excretion and in attempting to document exposure, it is
helpful to get an initial urine within 24 hours after

exposure. Since measurements are done in ppm, there is
no need for 24 hour urine collections unless one is interested in documenting the exact amount of excretion.

In addition to routine blood and urines for CBC, urin-
alysis and chemical screening, studies should be directed
at muscle enzymes such as aldolase, CPK and possibly iso-
enzymes of LDH. Myoglobinuria should also be considered.
In the event of central nervous system findings, a lumbar
puncture needs to be performed to rule out the possibility of an aseptic meningitis from any cause or evidence
of acute demyelinization. X-rays of the abdomen may be
valuable to rule out obstruction - which should not be
present. Nerve conduction studies will not be helpful
in the acute episode but should be performed following
the initial crisis in order to have baseline studies as
a means of following any possible future changes. Because of the possibility of myocardial changes, a baseline electrocardiogram should be performed early. In
the event of respiratory depression, blood gases would
be helpful in determining the need for assisted ventil-
ation.

Summary of Clinical Symptoms and Signs

Acute: Based upon the above reports, it appears that
a clinical syndrome of acute intoxication can occur following both dermal and gastrointestinal absorption and
that the dosage may be small. The principal symptoms
are nausea, abdominal pain and diarrhea. Neurological
symptoms are weakness, paresthesias and diminished coordination. Signs are evidence of hypermotility of the
gastrointestinal tract without evidence of any type of
obstruction, muscle fibrillation, decreased coordination,
diminished vibratory and proprioceptive sensation, and
diminished or absent deep tendon reflexes but with the
presence of superficial reflexes. Cranial nerves should
be intact.

Chronic: There are no known cases of chronic illness
developing insidiously and progressively from 2,4-D.
Following acute illness, neurological symptoms and signs
may persist for years but are not known to be exacerbated
with re-exposure.

Specific Therapy and Follow-up

   In the patient who has ingested 2,4-D, the usual procedure of attempting to empty the gastrointestinal tract
is necessary. If the patient is alert and emesis has not
occurred, Syrup of Ipecac should be utilized. If the
consciousness level is depressed, the stomach should be
intubated and aspiration and lavage performed. It is
important to determine whether the carrier is a petroleum
solvent since this increases the need to prevent pulmonary aspiration. In this case, it would be wise to in-
tubate the trachea prior to the stomach. Following aspiration, the stomach should be lavaged with isotonic
saline or sodium bicarbonate and then activated charcoal
should be administered. A cathartic may be given to
promote passage through the gastrointestinal tract.
   In the patient in whom absorption is known to have
already occurred, fluid intake should be increased via
intravenous fluids in order to accelerate renal excretion.
Central nervous system symptoms and/or signs may be treated symptomatically with diazepam.
   Laboratory evaluation and follow-up should be performed as described in the section under human toxicology.
   A most instructive case of treatment of 2,4-D intoxication, combined with mecoprop, has been reported by
Prescott, Park and Darrien (1979). In this case, a man
tried to poison himself with a weed killer containing
16.1% 2,4-D and 21.4% mecoprop. The plasma concentrations
on the man's admission were 335 and 400 mcg/ml respectively but the patient was fully conscious at the time. He
then gradually went into a deep coma. The plasma half-
life values of 2,4-D and mecoprop were measurable at 143
and 40 hours respectively. At this time, the mean urine
pH was 5.74. Over 90% of the 2,4-D excreted was recovered in the urine in an unchanged form. With the patient's
condition deteriorating, forced alkaline diuresis was
started using sodium bicarbonate intravenously. Rapid
diuresis occurred with excretion of 2,4-D. The patient
had other laboratory work performed during the severe
acute illness showing evidence of hemoglobinuria and
severe myopathy or myotonia with elevated CPK and LDH
values but with normal alkaline phosphatase and bili-
rubins. Electrocardiographic changes consisted of T wave
inversions and sinus tachycardia. Initial electrolytes
demonstrated a severe metabolic acidosis. The patient's
recovery was complete and apparently he had no residual
effect although the estimated ingested dose was very

large with total amounts of 2,4-D and mecoprop recovered
in the urine being 6.66 and 7.64 grams respectively.
Thus, the patient must have absorbed 70 ml of the concentrated weed killer. With alkaline diuresis, the plasma
biological half-life of the 2,4-D rapidly fell to 3.7
hours. The excretion increased rapidly when the urinary
pH was above 7.0. The effects on the plasma concentrations of the mecoprop were less dramatic but half-life
values did improve from 24 to 11 hours. In this case,
the patient regained consciousness four days after ingestion when the plasma concentration of 2,4-D and mecoprop had reached about 100 mcg/ml.

Dioxin

The polychlorinated dibenzo-p-dioxins (PCDDs) are
presently the subject of widespread public and scientific
curiosity and debate. A similar class of chemicals, the
polychlorinated dibenzofurans (PCDFs) are also occasional
contaminants in a variety of chemicals, although this
class will not be discussed here. The basic chemical
structure of the PCDDs and PCDFs is shown below.

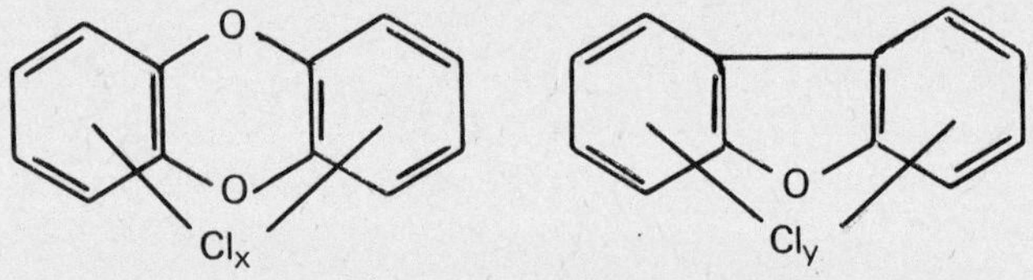

Although the lay press frequently used the term "Dioxin"
when referring to a specific compound of this class,
there are known to be a large number of potential isomers
which have a considerable range in toxicology. The most
controversial of these is the 2,3,7,8-tetrachlorodibenzo-
p-dioxin, commonly referred to as TCDD, which is a manufacturing contaminant in the production of 2,4,5-T,
trichlorophenol and hexachlorobenzene. A list of the
possible isomers is shown below.

Chlorine atoms	PCDD isomers	PCDF isomers
1	2	4
2	10	16
3	14	28
4	22	38
5	14	28
6	10	16
7	2	4
8	1	1
Total	75	135

Animal Toxicology Studies

In acute lethal dose experiments, the toxicity of the various PCDD isomers has striking variation, with the most toxic isomer being the 2,3,7,8 form. McConnell (1978) has summarized this material and it is presented below.

The following discussion on the specific toxic effects of TCDD has been summarized by the IARC (1978).

Animal toxicology studies are most extensive with the 2,3,7,8-tetrachlorodibenzo-p-dioxin since this chemical is not only known to be present in some agricultural chemicals but is the most potent of all the PCDDs. The toxic effects are known to vary considerably in different species of animals, as shown in the table from McConnell. In the monkey, McNulty (1977) stated that less than 1 ug/ kg body weight of TCDD was lethal to male rhesus monkeys. McConnell (1978) reported an LD_{50} in female rhesus monkeys as less than 70 ug/kg body weight.

TCDD has been found to be extremely toxic to monkeys. Allen and co-workers (1977) administered a diet with 500 parts per trillion of TCDD to eight adult female rhesus monkeys for nine months. The effects included acne, loss of hair and eyelashes and periorbital edema during the first three months of exposure. There was also a decrease in 17 beta-estradiol and progesterone levels as well as the development of irregularities in the monkey's menstrual cycles. The monkeys developed inability to conceive and early abortions occurred in the animals after six months exposure, although death also occurred in five of the eight experimental animals. Death was preceded by severe pancytopenia. Other find-

Estimated single oral lethal dose$_{50-30}$ values of certain polychlorinated dibenzo-p-dioxin isomers

Chlorine isomer	Guinea-pigs		Mice	
	ug/kg bw	u mole/kg bw	ug/kg bw	u mole/kg bw
2,8	>300,000	>1,180	-	-
2,3,7	29,444	120.41	>3,000	>10
2,3,7,8	2	0.006	283.7	0.88
1,2,3,7,8	3.1	0.009	337.5	0.94
1,2,4,7,8	1,125	3.15	>5,000	>14
1,2,3,4,7,8	72.5	0.185	825	2.11
1,2,3,6,7,8	70-100[c]	0.178-0.255	1,250	3.19
1,2,3,7,8,9	60-100[c]	0.153-0.255	>1,440	>3.67
1,2,3,4,6,7,8	600	>1.400	-	-
1-NO2-3,7,8	>30,000	>90	-	-
1-NH2-3,7,8	>30,000	>99	-	-
1-NO2-2,3,7,8	47.5	0.129	>2,000	>5.4
1-NH2-2,3,7,8	194.2	0.576	>4,800	>14.2

From: McConnell (1978)

ings included cardiac hypertrophy, edema, hyperplasia
and metaplasia of ductal tissue throughout the body,
hypertrophic gastritis and hepato-biliary changes.
Death was usually attributed to hemorrhage secondary
to severe thrombocytopenia.

The toxic syndromes produced by the PCDDs in experimental animals have been divided into six basic categories:

1. <u>Chloracne</u>: Chloracne is the principal outward
manifestation of intoxication from PCDD. Clasically, it
has the outward appearance of an acneform dermatitis and
originally received this name in clinical medicine because the acne appeared after exposure to chlorinated
chemicals. The typical classical chloracne has specific
histological characteristics, namely the development of
hyperkeratinization, i.e. keratin cyst formation is the
mechanism for producing pustules or papules, as opposed
to the more characteristic inflammatory lesion of acne
vulgaris. A number of PCDDs have been shown to produce
chloracne in experimental animals, with the major chemicals responsible being the tetrachlorodioxins, the hexa-
chlorodioxins and the heptachlorodioxins. In addition to
PCDDs, it is also known that the PCDFs may cause chloracne.

When appearing in human beings, chloracne usually
occurs several weeks or more after expousre begins and is
dose dependent. Upon the development of this disease,
the changes in the skin are usually prolonged and are
reported to last two to three years after exposure has
ceased. There is no specific treatment other than careful attention to good skin hygiene and possibly the use
of keratolyzing agents. Upon clearing, the common manifestation is to have areas of hypopigmented or hyperpig-
mented scarring and atrophy.

In human beings, it is important to recognize that
chloracne does not characteristically involve the face,
neck and upper shoulders as acne vulgaris but rather may
also involve the areas of the scalp, axilla and torso.
In other words, it is much more generalized than typical
acne vulgaris.

In all reports of chronic intoxication from tetra-
dioxins, chloracne has appeared in no less than 75% of
cases.

2. <u>Hepatotoxicity</u>: The liver is clearly a very susceptible organ to PCDDs and the degree of hepatic involve-

ment appears to be dose-dependent. There is considerable
variation in animal susceptibility with guinea-pigs and
monkeys being the most susceptible. In addition to hepatic changes ranging from stimulation of smooth endoplasmic reticulum to frank hepatic necrosis, a specific
enzyme change which is noticeable leads to the production
of hepatic porphyria. Hepatic porphyrin accumulation has
been observed in mice, rats, and chickens. In human
beings, long-term exposure to TCDD has been associated
with the syndrome of porphyria cutanea tarda. This is
a skin disease characterized by varying degrees of erythema, fissures, bullae or vesicle formation, scaling
and/or exfoliation. Although primarily a dermatological
condition, it may be associated with the development of
neuropsychiatric signs. Studies which are still in an
early developmental stage would indicate that there may
be changes of porphyrin metabolism associated with
populations exposed to chlorinated hydrocarbons in
general (Strik, 1978).

3. Hypoplasia of the Lymphoid Tissues and/or Bone
Marrow: Hypoplasia of the thymus gland has been observed
in mice, rats, guinea-pigs and monkeys with the most
significant findings occurring in both mice and guinea-
pigs treated with sublethal dosages of TCDD. A series of
articles by Vos (1978) have demonstrated changes in cell-
mediated immunity as a principal finding at levels which
did not produce overt clinical or pathological changes,
e.g. 1 mg/kg body weight given to mice orally once weekly
for four weeks.
Hematological changes can be seen at relatively high
dosages in a number of animals but the significance of
this finding may be one of direct toxicity rather than
any selective type of depletion of the lymphoid system.
Again, the monkey is a very susceptible animal and chronic feeding experiments at levels of 2-3 mcg TCDD have
shown extensive pancytopenia (Allen, 1977).

4. Embryo Toxicity and Teratogenicity of 2,3,7,8-
Tetrachlorodibenzo-p-dioxin: This subject has received
more public attention than any other aspect of this chemical and was the major consideration behind the recent
temporary restriction of the use of 2,4,5-T by the Environmental Protection Agency in March, 1979. In repeated
or single dosages of 2,3,7,8-tetrachlorodibenzo-p-dioxin
in mice, as little as 1-10 mcg/kg body weight causes increased frequency of cleft palate and kidney abnormalit-

ies (Courtney and Moore, 1971). In rats, embryo-lethal effects occur under experimental conditions (Sparschu, 1970 and 1971). Foetal kidney abnormalities have also been shown to occur and may progress into a hydronephrosis during the postnatal period (Moore, 1973). Other effects, such as intestinal hemorrhage, fatty generation of fetal livers or the development of subcutaneous edema in feeding experiments, are not considered to be teratogenic but are rather the direct result of toxic levels of fetal exposure. In teratogenic studies on rodents, Sparschu found the lowest effective dose to be 1.25 mcg/kg/day. In studying mice and rats, Courtney and Moore found that a dose of 1 mcg/kg/day was required to produce kidney malformations and that cleft palate in mice appeared at about 3 mcg/kg/day.

The continuous administration of 0.001 mcg/kg/day to male and female rats for 90 days prior to mating and through weaning of offspring produced no effect on fertility according to studies by Murray (1979). The above study continued through three generations, with each preceeding generation sacrificed at weaning of its offspring. The third generation was maintained until two years from the beginning of treatment of the first generation. Toxicity and poor litter survival forced termination of feeding at 0.1 mcg/kg/day and 0.01 mcg/kg/day caused decreased fertility in the first and second generations. In the second and third generation litters, the animals were smaller, and growth and survival were decreased after treatment of 0.01 mcg/kg/day.

Murray, et al (1979) have performed three generation rat reproduction studies with TCDD and have demonstrated that the ingestion of 0.1 mg/kg/day decreased both fertility and litter survival in the F_0 generation. Exposure to 0.01 mg/kg/day decreased fertility in the F_1 and F_2 generations but not in the F_0 generation.

Arising from the concern of Vietnam veterans' exposure to Agent Orange and the possibility of effects upon human reproduction, a study was recently completed by Lamb, et al (1980) to determine the effect of mixtures of a simulated Agent Orange on reproduction and fertility of treated male mice. The male mice were given feed containing varying concentrations with a maximum daily dose given of approximately 40 mg/kg 2,4-D, 40 mg/kg 2,4,5-T and 2.5 mcg/kg of TCDD. At the conclusion of an eight week dosing period, treated males were mated. Mating frequency, average fertility, percent implantation and resorption sites and percent fetal malformation were all measured in relation to the treatment. No significant decrease in fertility or reproduction was noted. There was no evidence of germ cell toxicity as measured by sperm concentration, motility, and percent sperm abnormalities. Survival of offspring and neonatal development was apparently unaffected by paternal exposure to the simulated mixture of Agent Orange or the concentration of 2,4-D, 2,4,5-T and TCDD as described above.

From a standpoint of classical toxicology analysis, it should be noted that the teratogenic potential of a chemical is usually considered in two ways: the first is the absolute dose of the chemical given to the pregnant animal on a body weight basis - which in the case of TCDD is extremely low; the second method of relating teratogenic potential is to compare the dose required for teratogenic effect with the dose needed to produce general toxic effect in the mother. Most toxicologists believe that a realistic approach to relating teratogenic potential of a chemical is to utilize both the absolute dose and the relationship of dosage to toxic effects. For example, if a chemical has a very low absolute dose to produce a teratogen, it may not necessarily be looked upon as a strong teratogen if at the same time it also produces illness in the mother, or, produces illness at a level which is fairly close to the teratogenic dose. At the least, one can say that given a chemical in which the teratogenic and the acute or chronic toxic dose are fairly close, one should expect to see illness in the mothers as well as teratogenic effects in the fetus. Specifically in relation to TCDD, this chemical is known to have an extremely low absolute teratogenic dose but, at the same time, its teratogenic potential may be "weak" because the dose required to produce teratogenesis is very close to that required to produce general toxic effects in the mother. For example, in the guinea-pig, TCDD teratogenesis has not been studied because the teratogenic dose is apparently higher than the lethal dose.

5. Chick Edema Disease: A syndrome of hydroparacardium, ascites, subcutaneous edema, liver necrosis and death has been described in chickens following the administration of toxic fats which were later identified to be commercial oleic and stearic acids produced from inedible tallow recovered from animal hides. The animal hides had been treated with trichlorophenols and pentachlorophenols in the process of curing. The edema causative factor was discovered to be a mixture of hexa-, tetra- and octa-

Summary of the toxic effects of
2,3,7,8-tetrachlorodibenzo-p-dioxin

	Mice	Guinea-pigs	Monkey (female)
Thymus involution	+++	+++	+++

Spleen
  reduction
  (white pulp)
	+	+	+

Bone marrow hypoplasia	±	++	+

Liver
  megalocytosis/
    degeneration
	+++	−	−

Bile duce hyperplasia	±	±	+++
Testicular degeneration	++	+++	NA
Renal pelvis hyperplasia	−	++	+
Urinary bladder hyperplasia	−	++	−

Adrenal
  cortical atrophy
  (Zona Glomerulosa)
	−	++	−

Haemorrhage
  intestinal
  adrenal
	+
	−
		+
		++
			−
			−

Ascites	++	−	+
Cutaneous lesions	−	−	+++

NA= not applicable

dioxins (Cantrell, 1969 and Firestone, 1973). Similar edematous effects have also been observed in rats, pigs, dogs and monkeys.

6. <u>Enzyme Induction</u>: A number of enzyme activities, most notably from the liver, can be stimulated by exposure to a variety of the dioxins. These enzymes are principally microsomal drug metabolizing enzymes and intoxication with the dioxins results in a marked increase in the cellular smooth endoplasmic reticulum content of both hepatic and renal cells. Some specific enzymes which are known to be affected are the steroid-hormone-metabolizing enzyme systems, glutathione-S transferase, delta-amino levulinic acid synthetase and aryl hydrocarbon hydroxylase.

Mutagenicity

The mutagenicity of the dioxin compounds has been reviewed by Wassom (1977). This material is reviewed by the working group of the NIEHS/IARC (1978) and is quoted below.

"Only four dioxin isomers have been evaluated for mutagenicity: the 2,7-di-, 2,3,7,8-tetra-, and the octa-CDDs as well as the unsubstituted dibenzo-p-dioxins.

"2,3,7,8-tetra-CDD increased the reversion frequency to streptamycin independence in <u>Escherichia coli</u> Sd-4. In <u>Salmonella typhimurium</u>, frameshift mutations in strain TA1532, but not base substitutions in strain TA1530, were induced by toxic concentrations of 2,3,7,8-tetra-CDD. In plate assays, the response was positive with <u>S. typhimurium</u> TA1532, doubtful with TA1531 and TA1534, and negative with G46 and TA1530. McCann tested 2,3,7,8-tetra-CDD in <u>S. typhimurium</u> both with and without metabolic activation, using a spot-test and the standard plate test with strains TA1532, TA1535, TA1537 and TA1538; all these tests were negative

Octa-CDD was non-mutagenic in <u>S. typhimurium</u> strains G46, TA1530 and TA1531, and doubtful results were obtained with strains TA1532 and TA1534. Metabolic activation systems were not

included in any of these microbiological
assays.

"Inhibition of mitosis and chromosomal
abnormalities (dicentric bridges and chro-
matin fusion with formation of multinuclei
or a single large nucleus) were observed
in endosperm cells of the African blood
lily (Haemanthus Katherinae Baker) treated
with 2,3,7,8-tetra-CDD in the presence
or absence of 2,4,5-T.

"No chromosomal aberrations were observed
in bone-marrow cells of male rats treated
with 2,7-di-CDD, 2,3,7,8-tetra-CDD, or
dibenzo-p-dioxin by oral intubation, with
2,3,7,8-tetra-CDD by intraperitoneal injection or orally. However, when Osborne
Mendel rats of both sexes were treated
twice weekly for 13 weeks with 2,3,7,8-
tetra-CDD, a significant but weak increase
in the number of chromosome aberrations
in bone marrow cells was reported.

"2,3,7,8-tetra-CDD did not induce dominant lethal mutations in Wistar rats after
oral administration to males for seven
days."

Evidence that TCDD is a mutagen is inconclusive and
is weakened by studies demonstrating that TCDD does not
bind with DNA and that it has very poor covalent binding
capacity. The latter, i.e. the ability of the compound
to be electrophilic, is considered to be of major importance for the chemical to be a mutagen. In the case of
TCDD, the binding capacity is four to six orders of magnitude lower than that observed with most chemical carcinogens (Poland and Glover, 1979). In addition, Pitot
and coworkers (1980) have demonstrated that TCDD is a
promoter of carcinogenesis and not an initiator. Again,
it is likely that most mutagenic chemicals are initiators
or complete carcinogens rather than promoters.

In summary, it would appear that TCDD is a weak mutagen.

Carcinogenicity of TCDD

There are three published reports indicating that the
chronic administration of low levels of TCDD to rats is

associated with an increased incidence of neoplasia.
The first of these is the report by Van Miller, et al
(1977) and is summarized below by the IARC Report (1978).

"Groups of 10 male Sprague-Dawley rats
were fed a diet containing 2,3,7,8-tetra-
CDD for 78 weeks in the following amounts
(figures in parentheses are approximate
weekly doses): 1 part per trillion (0.0003
mcg/kg bw), 5 ppt (0.001), 50 ppt (0.01),
500 ppt (0.1), 1 part per billion (0.4),
5 ppb (2.0), 50 ppb (24), 500 ppb (240),
and 1000 ppb (500). The three highest
dose levels (50, 500 and 1000 ppb) were
toxic and killed all animals by the fourth
week. Of the six remaining test groups,
the overall incidence of neoplasms was
23/60 (38%); none occurred in the 1 ppt
group. In the 5 ppt group, 5/10 animals
had 6 neoplasms (ear-duct carcinoma, lymphocytic leukemia, adenocarcinoma, malignant
histocytoma (with metastases), angiosarcoma,
Leydig-cell adenoma). The following groups
also showed neoplasms: 50 ppt, 3 observed
in 3/10; 500 ppt, 4 observed in 4/10; 1 ppb,
5 observed in 4/10; 5 ppb, 10 observed in
7/10. Neoplasms were not observed in the
controls."

The above experimental data is interesting for several
reasons. At the three highest dosage levels, the experiment, of course, has no validity. In the six remaining
test groups, the incidence of neoplasm remains almost at
a plateau in the groups of 5 ppt (0.001 mcg/kg) through
5 ppb (2.0 mcg/kg). This would seem to indicate the
following possibilities: 1) absence of threshold, 2) an
as yet unknown secondary factor playing a role in the
development of neoplasia, and 3) error in experimental
method.
The work by Kociba (1978) is summarized as follows:

"Groups of 100 Sprague-Dawley rats (50
males and 50 females) received for two years
diets containing 0, 22, 210, and 22,000
parts per trillion (ppt), equivalent to
0.0, 0.001, 0.01, and 0.1 mcg 2,3,7,8-
tetra-CDD/kg bw/day. Continuous ingestion
of 0.001 mcg/kg bw/day did not cause any

chemically-related changes in tumour incidence
or toxicity; feeding with 0.01 mcg/kg bw/day
induced an increased incidence ($P<0.05$) of
hepatocellular hyperplastic nodules (females:
18/50 versus 8/86), of focal alveolar hyperplasia in the lungs, and of urinary excretion
of porphyrins (female). Dietary intake of
0.1 mcg/kg bw/day caused an increased incidence
($P<0.05$) of hepatocellular carcinomas (female:
11/49 versus 1/86) and squamous-cell carcinomas
of the lung (female: 7/49 versus 0/86), of
the hard palate/nasal turbinates (male:
3/50 versus 0/85), Further increased were
adenoma of the adrenal cortex (male) and
hepatocellular hyperplastic nodules (female).
At this dose, certain age-related lesions
were reduced (males: acinar adenoma of the
pancreas; females: granulosal cell neoplasm
of the ovary, benign and malignant tumours
of the mammary gland, pituitary adenoma,
and benign tumours of the uterus). Also
chronic administration of 2,3,7,8-tetra-CDD
caused multiple toxicologic effects, including
increased mortality, decreased body weight
gain, slight depression of certain hematologic
parameters, increased urinary excretion
of porphyrins and delta-aminolevulinic acid,
increased serum levels of alkaline phosphatase,
glutamyl transferase and serum glutamic
pyruvic transferase and morphologic changes
primarily of the hepatic, lymphoid, respiratory
and vascular tissues of the body."

The above report differs from that of Van Miller in
dosage and also is interesting because of the decrease
in some types of spontaneously occurring tumors.

The third report is that by Pitot (1980) showing TCDD
as a promotor.

Excepting for a controversial and preliminary report
by Tung (1973), there are no reports on humans indicating
that exposure to TCDD will cause an increased amount of
cancer in the general population. In most cases, studying the general public is an unsatisfactory method because of the huge number of variables and, therefore,
studies are undertaken on the severely occupationally
exposed worker. These studies are not conclusive because
of the length of time since known exposure occurred or

because of the number of individuals in the studies.
However, a report by Zack and Suskind (1980) showed no
increase in cancer mortality in proven cases of acute
TCDD intoxication after 30 years. The results of long-
term studies of industrial TCDD accidents are summarized
in the accompanying table.

Dioxins in 2,4-D

A study by Cochrane and co-workers (1980) on 16 samples
of 2,4-D esters and amines, representing the current
Canadian supplies, were analyzed for the presence of
different chlorinated dibenzo-p-dioxins. Eight of nine
ester and four of seven amine samples were found to contain di-, tri-, and tetra-chlorodibenzo-p-dioxin, although the ester formulations showed significantly higher
levels of contamination than the amine formulations. The
tetra-chlorodioxin observed was the 1,3,6,8 isomer and
there was no evidence of the 2,3,7,8 isomer present. An
additional 10 2,4,-D technical assay samples from four
different sources did not contain any mono-, di-, tri-,
or tetra-chlorodioxin at the lowest limit of detection
(1 ppb). Based simply upon acute toxic effects, the
three dioxins found in 2,4-D would be in a range of
15,000 times to one million times less acutely toxic than
2,3,7,8-TCDD. Other studies than acute toxicity will be
required.
Seemingly in anticipation of the expected finding that
a dichlorodibenzo-p-dioxin (DCDD) would be present as a
contaminant in 2,4-D, the National Cancer Institute Carcinogenesis Testing Program did make a report available
in 1979 on the carcinogenicity of this specific dioxin.
Under the conditions of the bioassay, DCDD was not carcinogenic for rats nor in a female strain of mice. A
marginal increased incidence of combinations of leukemias
and lymphomas, of hemangiosarcomas and hemangiomas, and
of hepatocullular carcinomas and adenomas in male mice
provided evidence that further studies should be performed.

Pharmacokinetics

The dioxins as a class are lipophilic. Following
absorption and distribution, it is believed that TCDD is
accumulated primarily in the liver, the kidneys and the

Long Term Studies of TCDD Accidents

Town and Country	Year	Number of Exposed Persons	Clinical Follow-up	Preliminary Observations
Nitro, WV, USA	1949	228	30 years	No significant effect to date
Ludwigshafen/ Rhein, Germany	1953	75	Mortality study – 24 years on all persons	6 cancer deaths to date (3 of stomach)
Amsterdam, Holland	1963	106	93 persons followed	8 deaths with 5 or 6 from cardiovascular disease
Bolsover, Derbyshire, UK	1968	90	50% still employed	1 death from myocardial infarction
Seveso, Italy	1976	40,000(?)	80-90%	Chloracne, possible transient hepatomegaly
Czechoslovakia	1965–1969	80	55 persons	5 deaths (2 CA, 1 CV, 1 cirrhosis). Possible high frequency of hyperlipidemia and hypertension

fat. It is not known whether TCDD is actively metabolized in the body. There appears to be conflicting evidence as to this point. A study by Allen (1977) on
primates indicates that, unlike the behavior of other
chlorinated hydrocarbons in fasted or underfed animals,
TCDD may not be lost from adipose tissue under conditions
which should lead to fat mobilization, such as starvation.

The half-life of TCDD residues in the body has been
determined, however, and experiments indicate it is in
the range of 16-31 days. The concentration of TCDD apparently reaches a maximum at a given dose rate. That
is, experiments by Fries and Marrow (1975) and also by
Rose (1976) have demonstrated that in long-term feeding
experiments, the retention approached a steady state
which would be approximately 10 times that of the daily
intake.

Tissue Distribution: Firestone and others (1973)
investigated tissue distribution and absorption of the
hexa-, hepta-, and octa-chlorodibenzo-p-dioxins in White
Leghorn chicks fed a diet containing 3% toxic fat or the
equivalent amount of unsaponifiable fraction isolated
from the toxic fat. Over 90% of the ingested higher
chloro-dioxins were excreted. No octa-chloro-dioxin
could be detected in the tissue analyses. Both the hexa-
and the hepta-chloro-dioxins were found in a variety of
tissues such as bone, heart, intestine, kidney, liver and
skin and alterations in the relative levels of the hexa-
and hepta-chloro-dioxins suggested that some of the
chloro-dioxins may be metabolized by the chick. In all
cases, the hexa-chloro-dioxin was the major higher
chloro-dioxin found and only a low level of one of the
hepta-chloro-dioxins was evident. The lower forms of
chlorinated dioxins (five chlorine or less) were not
examined in the above study.

When given over long periods of time, TCDD may not be
as toxic in experimental animals as when given in the
acute, single administration experiments. For example,
in studies where 400 mcg/kg (about 20 times the LD_{50}) of
TCDD were administered, liver concentrations approached
3.6 ppm (Van Miller, 1977). Kociba (1976) caused discernible, but minor, hepatic lesions at a total dose of
0.65 mcg/kg given over a period of seven weeks. The
expected concentration of TCDD in the liver at this intake should have been on the order of 20 ppb and a 10-
fold lower dose caused no histopathological damage.
This "adaptation" in long-term feeding experiments has

been used as an explanation for the lack of histopathological lesions found in beach mice that had accumulated
over 1,000 ppt of TCDD in their livers with studies performed at Eglin Air Base (Young, 1978).

Dioxins in the Environment

One of the most important, persistent, and nagging
problems of our times is to determine whether the dioxins
persist and accumulate in the environment. Initial emphasis has been placed upon the established fact that the
dioxins appear to be industrial contaminants and, therefore, pollutants. Because of the inherent extreme toxicity of some of the compounds and the unresolved questions relating to carcinogenesis and mutagenesis, etc.,
the environmental fate is a significant issue. Indeed,
much of the public, as well as the scientific population,
is polarized on this issue.

As for the dioxins being a natural chemical, it seems
likely that some of the isomers do occur naturally and
part of the question to be resolved is whether or not the
extremely toxic isomers are also naturally occurring
chemicals. There is evidence that pyrolysis (burning)
leads to the formation of dioxin class chemicals. Thus
the assertion that the dioxins have been around since the
beginning of fire and that these chemicals will never be
eliminated from nature. These findings have not been
totally accepted since one of the problems is, of course,
to determine the source of the dioxin from the burning
materials. In this regard, however, it is interesting to
note that a number of studies in other countries have
partially substantiated the finding that dioxins are
formed with burning since a number of different types of
dioxins, as well as dibenzofurans, are formed and can be
found in the fly ash of incinerators. (Smith, 1978;
Ahling, 1977; Buser, 1978 and Olie, 1977).

In the commercial world, the principal source of
dioxin is as TCDD contamination in chemicals such as
2,4,5-T. Initially, this herbicide contained 20-30
parts per million of TCDD although the chemical has now
been cleaned-up to contain a maximum of 0.02 ppm. A
point to be made is that "Agent Orange" is a good deal
different from the present formulation of commercial
2,4,5-T. In agriculture, when 2,4,5-T is applied at two
pounds per acre, a little less than 20 mcg of TCDD per
acre will occur. This amount of TCDD on vegetation is

impossible to detect by present analytical methods, therefore, it is generally necessary to predict what might happen to the material by examining the existing laboratory data.

When mixed into soil, degradation is very slow with a half-life of about one year. However, TCDD deposited on leaves and exposed to direct sunlight degrades with a half-life of a little more than one hour. The ultra-violet type of degradation is dose dependent upon the nature of the solvent or the type of organic binding which has occurred with the TCDD. Present studies indicate that when TCDD is applied on soil, the half-life is about 50-55 hours (Crosby, 1977). Nevertheless, when the chemical gets below the immediate top surface, i.e. in the first 6-7 cm of top soil, such photodegradation will not occur and, therefore, biodegradation would be dependent upon bacteria and this might be a very slow process. Although exposure was massive - 1,000 pounds per acre - TCDD persisted more than a decade in top soil at Eglin Air Force Base (Young, 1978).

In spite of limited solubility in water (0.2 ppb) studies by Matsumura and Benezet (1973) have shown that TCDD will accumulate in aquatic sediment and that lower organisms, such as shrimp and mosquito larvae, appear to concentrate TCDD. Because of the unusual early high concentration and the artificial method of getting the TCDD deposited upon the sediment, the significance of this accumulation has been questioned. Nevertheless, accumulation did occur. Similarly, given sufficient TCDD in an artificial situation where 162 ppb of TCDD was in water, concentrations of up to 879 ppb were later shown to be present in Daphnia. In experiments performed by Isensee and Jones (1975) at water concentrations of 7 ppt of TCDD, catfish accumulated concentrations of 100 ppb. This work has also been used to demonstrate that as soil or water concentrations decrease, so also do concentrations in the organisms of the system.

In contrast to experimental laboratory studies, field studies of fish and mammals have provided evidence for both supporting and contradicting claims of TCDD accumulation in higher animals and also the role that the accumulation might play. In particular, the area of Eglin Air Force Base which was used as a training area received 2,4,5-T as "Agent Orange" on the order of 1,000 pounds per acre. Now, many years later, animals living in this area are shown to have very high levels of TCDD in livers, however, they do not demonstrate any pathological changes and this may be the "adaptation" alluded to earlier.

In samples taken from areas treated with 2,4,5-T in a more normal fashion, no TCDD has been found in cow's milk or in beef fat of range-fed animals. TCDD has been found in beef fat at levels of 20.3 ppt in a controlled field experiment where 2,4,5-T was used at four pounds per acre. Again, this data is extremely arguable and is contramanded principally by other wild animal samples in treated forest areas of Western Oregon in which no concentrations of TCDD have been found. Analysis of human milk samples by Meselson and O'Keefe (1978) had initially suggested that some samples from San Angelo, Texas and from Oregon contained levels of 1-3 ppt of TCDD. However, this data has not been accepted as valid and has essentially been refuted. At this time, TCDD has not been found in human tissue with the exception of autopsy studies from Seveso, Italy - to be discussed next.

The Seveso, Italy Incident

On July 10, 1976, a reactor in a plant producing trichlorophenol as a preliminary step for later production of the antibacterial agent, hexachlorophene, had an exothermic-type (heat-forming) explosion resulting in the release of the contaminant TCDD into the local environment. The incident, occurring in a suburb of Milan called Seveso, has become an international cause celebre for both chemical adversaries and chemical advocates. Some magnitude of the severity of the environmental contamination can be assessed by considering that as much TCDD was released into a small community of approximately 750 square acres as is released in the entire continental United States per annum. From the very beginning, the incident has been controversial. The local authorities were notified of an accident within two days of the event, however, the evacuation of families did not begin until the 27th of July and was not completed for three to three and a half weeks after the explosion occurred. In the interim, assessment was made of the TCDD levels in the immediate environment. The area downwind from the plant was divided into three zones, based upon the severity of the TCDD contamination. In Zone A, the most heavily contaminated, a population of 736 people were fully evacuated. A population of 4,699 people lived in Zone B and women in their first trimester of pregnancy were advised to move out and children in the area were removed during the daylight

hours. The remaining zone, labelled Zone R, had a population of 31,800 people but since their contamination was
believed to be only minimal, the zone was considered an
area for respectful watching and the residents were not
moved but were placed under surveillance. For purposes
of health surveillance, the population of the surrounding
districts, totalling 220,000 people, were also placed
under surveillance by the local medical commission. TCDD
levels in Zones A, B and R were measured initially, however, earliest records of TCDD levels published are those
for December 1976, fully five months after the accident.
At this time, levels of TCDD for Zone A still averaged
230 mcg/m^2; in Zone B, measurement averaged 3.0 mcg/m^2
and in Zone R, measurements averaged 0-0.5 mcg/m^2. Because of the extreme danger to animal life, as well as
the expected danger to humans, the entire area of Zone A
was subjected to a lengthy "decontamination" proceeding,
the methodology of which has been discussed in other reviews. It is not the purpose of this document to review
the entire ecological implications of the Seveso incident.
For the interested reader, the position of the chemical
adversary can be found in papers by Whiteside (1977) and
by Commoner (1978). A neutral position can be found in
an article by Hay (1977).

The medical effects of the TCDD contamination in
Seveso have been most interesting to clinical, as well
as classical, toxicologists. Although argument is bound
to occur regarding methods of data collection and the
nature of evaluation and question of long-term problems,
it is apparent to everyone that the human being is a good
deal less susceptible to TCDD than is the experimental
animal. Unanswered problems clearly regard the future
development of cancer in the exposed population or possible mutagenic changes which will only be seen through
several generations.

The population was followed through a series of 11
parameters: 1) skin lesions (chloracne), 2) neurological
lesions, 3) functions of blood, liver and kidney systems,
4) growth of newborn and children, 5) rate of malformation (birth defects), 6) frequency of abortions, 7) cytogenetic anomalies, 8) immunological deficiency, 9) frequency of infectious diseases, 10) birth rate, and 11)
mortality rate. Some of these parameters are discussed
below. More complete detail can be found in the report
by Reggiani (1978a and 1978b) or by Homberger (1979).

Chloracne: This was the most striking clinical fea-
ture in all individuals. Children were particularly
susceptible, and in the Seveso area, repeated screenings
show that 0.6-1.2% of the examined population were affected to produce classical chloracne and up to 14% are
described as having possible chloracne. For most children, the lesions healed rapidly following removal from
the TCDD and, according to Homberger (1979), the second
screening performed on school children in April-May of
1977 revealed only a total incidence up to 0.4%. The
lesions appeared slowly, often beginning weeks to months
after the actual exposure occurred - a characteristic of
chronic TCDD intoxication. All told, there were a total
of 175 cases of confirmed chloracne - based upon clinical
examination - and a total of about 600 cases of possible
chloracne from the examination of the total population of
over 32,000 people. In the confirmed cases, chloracne
has been severe enough to persist in a large majority for
at least two years since the onset.

Neurological Lesions: A population of 224 children
and 625 adults were examined both clinically and by such
procedures as electromyography and motor conduction times.
Homberger (1979) describes no acute lesions of the peripheral or central nervous system but does describe the
gradual development of a peripheral neuritis which was
subclinical in terms of symptoms but definitive in terms
of the neuro-physiological examination. This 10% incidence of people with neuritis was found only in the heavily contaminated zone and no correlation could be demonstrated between the occurrence of chloracne and the
neurological findings. Interestingly, none of the children with chloracne had any impairment of nervous system
functions. Similarly, plant workers were also examined
for neurological changes and eight cases out of 156 were
found to have motor conduction impairment of a similar
nature to the general population. To date, no definitive
conclusions have been drawn as to the etiological relationship to the subclinical neuropathy with the TCDD
exposure.

Other Organ Involvement: There was no damage detected
of the hematopoietic or of the kidney systems. A transient hepatomegaly was described in about 8-10% of the
people examined and liver function studies showed a transient increase of serum transaminases and of gamma-GT in
about 10% of those people who were examined in Zone A and

Zone B. Again, interestingly, the plant workers had a lower incidence of abnormal liver function studies than the exposed population in Seveso. Preliminary reports indicate that there may be an increased level of delta-amino-levulinic acid excretion in the urine samples of the population. Further studies of this nature need to be performed. It has been proposed, although not yet proven, that there may not be a significant quantitative increase in the excretion of urinary porphyrins but that there may be a change in their proportions.

Abortions: The vexing problem of determining the number of spontaneous abortions occurring as the result of exposure has not been clearly answered as the result of Seveso. Many women went on to have therapeutic abortions and, therefore, the entire population at risk could not be sampled. The data collected indicate only that the number of spontaneous abortions was not higher than what would be expected in other parts of Italy or world-wide. The incidence of still births, spontaneous and induced abortions rate per number of calculated pregnancies for previous and post-years have been accumulated and are shown in the table below.

	Township	1973 %	1974 %	1975 %	1976 %	1977 %
Townships covering Zones A, B&R	Cesano	9.01	10.89	8.81	9.15	9.06
	Desio	15.54	13.43	13.58	8.91	14.54
	Meda	6.23	5.88	5.70	9.00	8.70
	Seveso	10.79	7.84	12.83	11.14	12.09
	Average	10.39	9.51	10.23	9.55	11.09
Townships outside contaminated zones	Barlassina	6.18	5.43	4.12	8.97	3.03
	Bovisio	9.46	11.05	14.61	12.82	16.56
	Lentate	1.82	1.85	1.87	1.59	5.85
	Muggio	11.45	13.72	9.86	12.67	14.38
	Nova M	13.44	15.03	11.72	15.36	12.64
	Seregno	13.28	11.09	9.85	8.75	12.07
	Varedo	10.30	9.09	11.36	7.02	10.34
	Average	9.41	9.60	9.05	9.59	10.69
	Seveso region	9.90	9.55	9.64	9.57	10.89

(World-wide: 15-20% - Lombardy region 12-15%)

Congenital Malformations: Probably the most controversial data collected from Seveso is that related to
congenital malformations. Examination of the data does
show a marked increase in the number of congenital malformations between 1976 and 1977, as demonstrated by the
following table showing the frequency of malformations in
the 11 districts of the Seveso zone.

| Year | Rate of malformations per 100 live-births | | |
	Number of live-births	Notified	Expected at the rate of 2.5-3%
1976 second semester	1417	4 (0.28%)	35-42
1977 12 months	2664	38 (1.42%)	66-80
1978 first quarter	684	5 (0.75%)	16-20

Regardless of changes in the reporting system, there is an
apparent increase in the percentage of malformations being
reported as compared to live births. For the chemical
advocate, this information is reassuring since the percentage is still below what would be predicted to occur
in the general population. For the chemical adversary,
the data collected is evidence that the chemical had a
profound effect upon the rate of congenital malformation
resulting in a significant increase. Further argument
exists because of the variety of malformations which were
observed. That is, based upon animal experiments, one
might only expect a high number of cleft palates or renal
disease. Instead, the neonatal malformations occurring
in Seveso were a wide variety of types. Again, the question is whether TCDD is so toxic that it could produce a
morphological heterogenecity. However, most embryologists
believe that a single causal agent (in this case TCDD)
should produce a congenital malformation of a fairly
homogeneous type. The accompanying table demonstrates
the variety of malformations which were seen.

Other Parameters: Examination of the embryo was performed on 34 cases of abortions and direct examination
did not detect any gross signs of abnormal development.
Histological examination on the aborted fetuses also was

Neonatal malformations in Seveso

Type and Pattern	1976	1977	1978 first quarter
Pulmonary aplasia	–	1	–
Anencephalia	–	1	–
Atresia of auditory meatus	–	1	–
Congenital cardiopathy	–	8	2
Vesical ectopia	–	1	–
Gastric extrophy	–	1	–
Hydrocephaly	–	1	–
Hypospadia	2	2	1
Abdominal malformation	–	2	–
Anal malformation	–	1	–
Pedalic malformation	–	10	–
Meningocele	–	1	–
Neoplasia	–	2	–
Defect osteogenesis	–	1	–
Down syndrome	2	2	–
Syndactyly	–	3	–
Cleft palate	–	–	1
Diaphragmatic hernia	–	–	1
Total	4	38	5

reported as normal. Chromosome analysis of maternal
peripheral blood, amniotic fluid cells and fetal tissues
were performed and were found to be within the accepted
standard frequency. Immunological studies, including
examination of serum immunoglobulins, complement, population of T and B lymphocytes, and reaction of T and B
lymphocytes to mitogens, were studied in 45 children from
Zone A, of which 20 had chloracne, and were compared
against 44 children who were not exposed to TCDD. No
significant difference could be found in the immune
responses of the groups studied. On the other hand, the
reported incidence of infectious disease rose from 435 in
1976 to 1219 in 1977 in the 11 township areas. This
seemingly contradicts the results of the basic immunological investigations. Chemical advocates believe the
increased infectious disease was the result of improved
reporting and awareness in the population, but does not
involve diseases where vaccination has been performed,

i.e. possibly strengthening the findings of a normal
immune response. Finally, the incidence of reported
infectious disease still did not exceed that of other
nearby communities in the province of Milan.

As stated earlier, the long-term questions such as
carcinogenicity and mutagenicity problems cannot be
ascertained at this time. Unfortunately, tissue samples
on human beings have not been routinely taken to date
from people involved in the Seveso accident. There is
one reported death from carcinoma of the pancreas in
which tissue samples showed levels of TCDD at concentrations of greater than 1 ppb with major concentration
occurring in the pancreas, liver, kidney and fat.

References

Ahling, B. and A. Lindskog (1977) Formation of polychlorinated dibenzo-p-dioxins and dibenzofurans during
combustion of a 2,4,5-T formulation. Chemosphere
8:461-468.

Aldred, J.E. (Chairman) (1978) Report of the Consultive
Council on Congenital Abnormalities in the Yarram
District. Minister of Health, Melbourne, Victoria,
Australia.

Allen, J.R., D.A. Barsotti, J.P. van Miller, L.J.
Abrahamson and J.J. Lalich (1977) Morphological
changes in monkeys consuming a diet containing low
levels of 2,3,7,8-tetrachlorodibenzo-p-dioxin.
Food Cosmet Toxicol 15:401-410.

Anderson, K.J., E.G. Leighty and M.T. Takahashi (1972)
Evaluation of herbicides for possible mutagenic
properties. J Agr Food Chem 20:649-656.

Axelson, O. and L. Sundell (1974) Herbicide exposure,
mortality and tumor incidence. An epidemiological
investigation on Swedish railroad workers. Work
Environ Health 11:21-28.

Axelson, O., C. Edling, H. Kling, K. Anderson, C.
Hogstedt and L. Sundell (1979) Updating the mortality
among pesticide exposed railroad workers.
Lakartigningen 76:3505-3506.

Bage, G., E. Cekanova and K.S. Larsson (1973) Teratogenic and embryotoxic effects of the herbicides di-
and trichlorophenoxyacetic acid (2,4-D and 2,4,5-T).
Acta Pharmacol Toxicol 32:408-416.

Berkley, M.C. and K.R. Magee (1963) Neuropathy following
exposure to a dimethylamine salt of 2,4-D. Arch
Intern Med 111:133-134.

Berwick, P. (1970) 2,4-Dichlorophenoxyacetic acid
poisoning in man. JAMA 214:1114-1117.

Bleiberg, J., M. Wallen, R. Brodkin and I.L. Applebaum
(1971) Industrially acquired porphyria. Arch
Dermatol 89:793-797.

Buser, H.R. and H.P. Bosshardt (1978) Identification of
polychlorinated dibenzo-p-dioxin isomers found in fly
ash. Chemosphere 2:165-172.

Cantrell, J.S., N.C. Webb and A.J. Mabis (1969)
Identification and crystal structure of hydropericar-
dium-producing factor; 1,2,3,7,8,9-hexachlorodibenzo-
p-dioxin. Acta Crystallogr, Sect B25:15-156.

Cochrane, W.P., J. Singh, W. Miles, B. Wakeford and J.
Scott (1980) Analysis of technical and formulated
products of 2,4-dichlorophenoxyacetic acid for the
presence of chlorinated dibenzo-p-dioxins. Presented
at the Workshop on the "Impact of Chlorinated Dioxins
and Related Compounds on the Environment, Rome, Italy,
October 22-24.

Collins, T.F.X. and C.H. Williams (1971) Teratogenic
studies with 2,4,5-T and 2,4-D in the hamster.
Bull Environ Contam Toxicol 6:559-567.

Commoner, B. (1978) Toxicologic time bomb. Hosp Prac
June, pp. 56-57.

Courtney, K.D. and J.A. Moore (1971) Teratology studies
with 2,4,5-trichlorophenoxyacetic acid and 2,3,7,8-
tetrachlorodibenzo-p-dioxin. Toxicol Pharmacol
20:396-403.

Crosby, D.C. and A.S. Wong (1977) Environmental
degradation of 2,3,7,8-tetrachlorodibenzo-p-dioxin
(TCDD). Science 195:1337-1338.

Davies, M.K. and R.T. Jung (1976) Lung involvement with
  "Verdone". Lancet 2:370.

Dost, F.N. (1977) Toxicology of phenoxy herbicides and
  hazard assessment of their use in reforestation.
  Task Force Report to the Oregon State University
  Environmental Health Sciences Center.

Dougherty, R.C. and K. Piotrowska (1976) Screening by
  negative chemical ionization mass spectrometry for
  environmental contamination with toxic residues:
  Application to human urines. Proc Natl Acad Sci USA
  73:1777-1781.

Drill, V.A. and T. Hiratzka (1953) Toxicity of
  2,4-dichlorophenoxyacetic acid and 2,4,5-trichloro-
  phenoxyacetic acid. Ind Hyg Occup Med 7:61-67.

Dudley, A.W.,Jr. and N.T. Thapar (1972) Fatal human
  ingestion of 2,4-D, a common herbicide. Arch Pathol
  94:270-275.

Environmental Protection Agency (1978) Rebuttable
  presumption against registration and continued
  registration of pesticide products containing 2,4,5-T.
  Fed Register 42:17116-17156.

Firestone, D., D.F. Flick, J. Ress and G.R. Higginbotham
  (1971) Distribution of chick edema factors in chick
  tissues. Jour AOAC 54:1293-1298.

Firestone, D. (1973) Etiology of chick edema disease.
  Environ Health 5:59-66.

Forest Service - USDA (1977) Pacific Northwest Region:
  Final Environmental Statement, Vegetation Management
  With Herbicides, Volume 1.

Fries, G.F. and G.S. Marrow (1975) Retention and
  excretion of 2,3,7,8-tetrachlorodibenzo-p-dioxin
  by rats. J Agr Food Chem 23:265-269.

Gehring, P.J., C.G. Kramer, B.A. Schwetz, J.Q. Rose and
  V.K. Rowe (1973) The fate of 2,4,5-trichlorophenoxy-
  acetic acid (2,4,5-T) following oral administration
  to man. Toxicol Appl Pharmacol 26:352-361.

Geldmacher-v. Mallinckrodt, M. and L. Lautenbach (1966)
Zwei todliche vergiftungen (suicid) mit chlorierten
phenoxyessigsauren (2,4-D und MCPS). Archiv Toxikol
21:261-278.

Goldstein, N.P., P.H. Jones and J.R. Brown (1959)
Peripheral neuropathy after exposure to an ester of
dichlorophenoxyacetic acid. JAMA 171:1306-1309.

Goulding, R.L., M.L. Montgomery and W.S. Staton (1972)
Waste pesticide management: Interim progress report.
Oregon State University, January 26.

Grolleau, G., E. de Lavaur and G. Siou (1974) Effets
du 2,4-D sur la reproduction des cailles et des
perdrix, apres application du produit par pulverisa-
tion sur les oeufs. Ann Zool Ecol Anim 6:313-331.

Hansen, W.H., M.L. Quaife, R.T. Habermann and O.C.
Fitzhugh (1971) Chronic toxicity of 2,4-dichloro-
phenoxyacetic acid in rats. Toxicol Appl Pharmacol
20:122-129.

Hardell, L. (1977) Malignant mesenchymal tumors and
exposure to phenoxy acids: A clinical observation.
Lakartidningen 74:2753-2754.

Hardell, L. and A. Sandstrom (1979) Malignant lymphoma
of histiocytic type and exposure to phenoxyacetic
acids or chlorophenols. Lancet 1:55-56.

Hardell, L., M. Eriksson and P. Lenner (1980) A case
control study: Malignant lymphomas and exposure to
chemicals, particularly organic solvents, chlorophenols, and phenoxy acids. Laekartidningen
77:208-210.

Hay, A.W.M. (1977) Tetrachlorodibenzo-p-dioxin release
at Seveso. Disasters 1:289-308.

Hill, E.V. and H. Carlisle (1947) Toxicity of 2,4-di-
chlorophenoxyacetic acid for experimental animals.
J Indust Hyg Toxicol 29:85-95.

Homberger, E., G. Reggiani, J. Sambeth and H. Wipf
(1979) The Seveso accident: Its nature, extent
and consequences. Ann Occup Hyg 22:327-367.

IARC (1978)   Long-term hazards of polychlorinated
dibenzodioxins and polychlorinated dibenzofurans.
International Agency For Research on Cancer Technical
Report #78/001, Lyon.

Innes, J.R.M., B.M. Ulland, M.G. Valerio, L. Petrucelli,
L. Fishbein, E.R. Hart, A.J. Pallotta, R.R. Bates,
H.L. Falk, J.J. Gart, M. Klein, I. Mitchell and
J. Peters (1969) Bioassay of pesticides and indus-
trial chemicals for tumorigenicity in mice: A
preliminary note.   J Natl Cancer Inst 42:1101-1114.

Isensee, A.R. and G.E. Jones (1975)   Distribution of
2,3,7,8-tetrachlorodibenzo-p-dioxin (TCDD) in
aquatic model ecosystem.   Environ Sci Technol
9:668-672.

Jensen, D. and L. Renberg (1976)   Distribution and
cytogenetic test of 2,4-D and 2,4,5-T phenoxyacetic
acids in mouse blood tissues.   Chem-Biol Interact
14:291-299.

Johnson, J.E. (1971)   The public health implications of
widespread use of the phenoxy herbicides and picloram.
Bioscience 21:899-905.

Kay, J.H., R.J. Palazzolo and J.C. Calandra (1965)
Subacute dermal toxicity of 2,4-D.   Arch Environ
Health 11:648-651.

Khera, K.S. and W.P. McKinley (1972)   Pre- and postnatal studies on 2,4,5-trichlorophenoxyacetic acid,
2,4-dichlorophenoxyacetic acid and their derivatives
in rats.   Toxicol Appl Pharmacol 22:14-28.

Kilian, D.J., M.C. Benge, R.V. Johnston and E.B.
Whorton, Jr. (1974) Cytogenetic studies of personnel
who manufacture 2,4,5-T. (Personal communication,
unpublished manuscript).

Kociba, R.J., D.G. Keyes, J.E. Beyer, R.M. Carreon,
C.E. Wade, D.A. Kittenber, R.P. Kalnins, L.E. Frauson,
C.N. Park, S.D. Barnard, R.A. Hummel and C.G. Humiston
(1978) Results of a two-year chronic toxicity and
oncogenicity study of 2,3,7,8-tetrachlorodibenzo-p-
dioxin in rats. Toxicol Appl Pharmacol 45:298.

Kohli, J.D., R.N. Khanna, B.N. Gupta, M.M. Dhar, J.G. Tandom and K.P. Sircar (1974) The fate of 2,4,5-trichlorophenoxyacetic acid (2,4,5-T following oral administration to man. Toxicol Appl Pharmacol 26:352-361.

Lamb, J.C., J.A. Moore and T.A. Marks (1980) Evaluation of 2,4-dichlorophenoxyacetic acid (2,4-D), 2,4,5-tri-chlorophenoxyacetic acid (2,4,5-T) and 2,3,7,8-tetra-chlorodibenzo-p-dioxin (TCDD) toxicity in C57BL/6 mice: Reproduction and fertility in treated male mice and evaluation of congenital malformations in their offspring. National Toxicology Program Publication #80-44, Research Triangle Park, NC 27709.

Lavy, T.L. (1978) Measurement of 2,4,5-T exposure of forest workers. Altheimer Laboratory, University of Arkansas.

Lavy, T.L. (1980) Determination of 2,4-D exposure received by forestry applicators, Spring 1980. National Forest Products Association.

Matsumura, A. (1970) The fate of 2,4,5-trichloro-phenoxyacetic acid in man. Sangyo Igaku 12:446-451.

Matsumura, F. and H.J. Benezet (1973) Studies on the bioaccumulation of microbial degradation of 2,3,7,8-tetrachlorodibenzo-p-dioxin (TCDD). Environ Health Perspect 5:253-258.

Meselson, M., P.W. O'Keefe and R. Baughman (1978) The evaluation of possible health hazards from TCDD in the environment. IN: Presentation For Symposium on the Use of Herbicides in Forestry, Arlington, VA.

Moore, J.A., B.N. Gupta, J.G. Zinkl and J.G. Vos (1973) Postnatal effects of maternal exposure to 2,3,7,8-tetrachlorodibenzo-p-dioxin (TCDD). Environ Health Perspect 7:81-85.

Muranyi-Kovacs, I., G. Rudali and J. Imbert (1976) Bioassay of 2,4,5-trichlorophenoxyacetic acid for carcinogenicity in mice. Brit J Cancer 33:626-633.

Murray, F.J., F.A. Smith, K.D. Nitschke, C.G. Humiston, R.J. Kociba and B.A. Schwetz (1979) Three-generation reproductive study of rats given 2,3,7,8-tetrachloro-dibenzo-p-dioxin (TCDD) in the diet. Toxicol Appl Pharmacol 50:241-252.

McConnell, E.E., J.A. Moore, J.K. Haseman and M.W. Harris (1978) The comparative toxicity of chlorinated dibenzo-p-dioxins in mice and guinea pigs. Toxicol Appl Pharmacol 44:335-356.

McNulty, W.P. (1977) Toxicity of 2,3,7,8-tetrachloro-dibenzo-p-dioxin for rhesus monkeys: Brief report. Bull Environ Contam Toxicol 18:108-109.

National Cancer Institute (1979) Bioassay of 2,7-di-chlorodibenzo-p-dioxin (DCDD) for possible carcino-genicity. Technical Report Series #123.

Nelson, C.J., J.F. Holson, H.G. Green and D.W. Gaylor (1979) Retrospective study of the relationship between agricultural use of 2,4,5-T and cleft palate occurrence in Arkansas. Teratology 19:377-384.

Nielsen, K., B. Kaempe and J. Jensen-Holm (1965) Fatal poisonings in man by 2,4-dichlorophenoxyacetic acid (2,4-D): Determination of the agent in forensic materials. Acta Pharmacol Toxicol 22:224-234.

Norris, L.A. (1967) Chemical brush control and herbicide residues in the forest environment. IN: Herbicides and Vegetation Management Symposium, Oregon State University, pp. 103-123.

Norris, L.A. (1969) Degradation of several herbicides in red alder forest floor material. Weed Soc for Weed Sci Res, Prog Rept, pp. 21-22.

Olie, K., P.L. Vermeulen and O. Hutzinger (1977) Chlorodibenzo-p-dioxins and chlorodibenzofurans are trace components of fly ash and flue gas of some municipal incinerators in the Netherlands. Chemosphere 6:455-459.

Ott, M.G., B.B. Holder and R.D. Olson (1980) A mortality analysis of employees engaged in the manufacture
of 2,4,5-trichlorophenoxyacetic acid. J Occup Med
22:47-50.

Pitot, H.C., T. Goldsworthy, H.A. Campbell and A. Poland
(1980) Quantitative evaluation of the promotion by
2,3,7,8-tetrachlorodibenzo-p-dioxin of hepatocarcino-
genesis from diethylnitrosamine. Cancer Res
40:3616-3620.

Poland, A.P., D. Smith, G. Metter and P. Possick (1971)
A health survey of workers in a 2,4-D and 2,4,5-T
plant. Arch Environ Health 22:316-327.

Poland, A. and E. Glover (1979) An estimate of the
maximum in vivo covalent binding of 2,3,7,8-tetra-
chlorodibenzo-p-dioxin to rat liver protein, ribosomal
RNA, and DNA. Cancer Res 39:3341-3344.

Prescott, L.F., J. Park and I. Darrien (1979) Treatment
of severe 2,4-D and Mecoprop intoxication with
alkaline diuresis. Br J Clin Pharmacol 7:111-116.

Randolph, T.G. (1976) Human Ecology and Susceptibility
to the Chemical Environment, Charles C. Thomas,
Springfield, IL.

Rea, W.J. (1977) Environmentally triggered small vessel
vasculitis. Ann Allergy 38:245-251.

Reggiani, G. (1978a) The estimation of the TCDD toxic
potential in the light of the Seveso accident.
Paper presented at the 20th Congress of the European
Society of Toxicology, West Berlin, June 25-28.

Reggiani, G. (1978b) Report of the Parlimentary
Commission of Inquiry into the escape of toxic
substances which took place on the 10th of June,
1976 in the Icmesa factory and into the potential
health risks and risks to the environment deriving
from industrial activity. Rome, July.

Rose, J.Q., J.C. Ransey, T.H. Wentzler, R.A. Hummel
and P.J. Gehring (1976) The fate of 2,3,7,8-tetra-
chlorodibenzo-p-dioxin following single and repeated
oral doses to the rat. Toxicol Appl Pharmacol
36:209-226.

Sauerhoff, M.W., W.H. Braun, G.E. Blau and P.J. Gehring
(1977) The fate of 2,4-dichlorophenoxyacetic acid
(2,4-D) following oral administration to man.
Toxicol 8:3-11.

Schwetz, B.A., G.L. Sparschu and P.J. Gehring (1971)
The effect of 2,4-dichlorophenoxyacetic acid (2,4-D)
and esters of 2,4-D on rat embryonal, foetal and
neonatal growth and development. Fd Cosmet Toxicol
9:801-817.

Seabury, J.H. (1963) Toxicity of 2,4-dichlorophenoxy-
acetic acid for man and dog. Arch Environ Health
7:202-209.

Seiler, J.P. (1979) Phenoxyacids as inhibitors of
testicular DNA synthesis in male mice. Bull Environ
Contam Toxicol 21:89-92.

Shapley, D. (1974) Herbicides: Academy finds damage in
Vietnam after a fight of its own. Science
183:1177-1180.

Smith, R.J. (1978) Dioxins have been present since the
advent of fire, says Dow. Science 202:1166-1167.

Sparschu, G.L., F.L. Dunn and V.K. Rowe (1970) Teratogenic study of 2,3,7,8-tetrachlorodibenzo-p-dioxin
in the rat. Toxicol Appl Pharmacol 17:317.

Sparschu, G.L., F.L. Dunn and V.K. Rowe (1971) Study
of the teratogenicity of 2,3,7,8-tetrachlorodibenzo-
p-dioxin in the rat. Food Cosmet Toxicol 9:405-412.

Strik, J.J.T.W.A. (1978) Porphyrins in urine as
indication for exposure to chlorinated hydrocarbons.
N.Y. Acad Sci, Sci Week.

Todd, R.L. (1962) A case of 2,4-D intoxication.
J Iowa Med Soc 52:663-664.

Tung, T.T. (1973) Primary cancer of the liver in
    Viet Nam. Chirurgie 99:427-436.

Van Miller, J.P., J.J. Lalich and J.R. Allen (1977)
    Increased incidence of neoplasms in rats exposed to
    low levels of 2,3,7,8-tetrachlorodibenzo-p-dioxin.
    Chemosphere 6:537-544.

Vos, J.G. (1978) 2,3,7,8-Tetrachlorodibenzo-para-
    dioxin: Effects and mechanisms. IN: Ramel, C. (ed),
    Chlorinated Phenoxy Acids and Their Dioxins: Mode of
    Action, Health Risks and Environmental Effects,
    Ecol Bull (Stockholm) 27:165-176.

Walker, E.M.,Jr., R.H. Gadsdan, L.M. Atkins and G.R.
    Gale (1972) Some effects of 2,4-D and 2,4,5-T on
    Ehrlich ascites tumor cells in vivo and in vitro.
    Indust Med 41:22-27.

Wassom, J.S., J.E. Huff and N. Loprieno (1977) A
    review of the genetic toxicology of chlorinated
    dibenzo-p-dioxins. Mutat Res 47:141-160.

Whiteside, T. (1977) A reporter at large: The pendulum
    and the toxic cloud. The New Yorker, July 25th,
    p.30.

Wiersma, G.B., H. Tai and P.F. Sand (1972) Pesticide
    residue levels in soils. Pest Monit J 6:194-228.

Woolson, E.A., R.F. Thomas and P.D.J. Ensor (1972)
    Survey of polychlorodibenzo-p-dioxin content in
    selected pesticides. J Agr Food Chem 20:351-354.

Yoder, J., M. Watson and W. Benson (1973) Lymphocyte
    chromosome analysis of agricultural workers during
    extensive occupational exposure to pesticides.
    Mutat Res 21:335-340.

Young, A.L., C.E. Thalken and D.D. Harrison (1978)
    Persistence, bioaccumulation and toxicology of TCDD
    in an ecosystem treated with massive quantities of
    2,4,5-T herbicide. Symposium on Avian and Mammalian
    Wildlife Toxicology, American Society for Testing
    Materials, New Orleans, LA, October 17th.

Zack, J.A. and R.R. Suskind (1980) The mortality
    experience of workers exposed to tetrachlorodibenzo-
    dioxin in a trichlorophenol process accident.
    J Occup Med 22:11-14.

Zetterberg, G, L. Busk, R. Elovson, I. Starec-Norden-
    hammer and H. Tyttman (1977) The influence of pH
    on the effects of 2,4-D (2,4-dichlorophenoxyacetic
    acid, Na salt) on Saccharomyces cerevisiae and
    Salmonella typhimurium. Mutat Res 42:3-18, 1977.

3

Dipyridyl Compounds–Paraquat

The dipyridyl chemicals are a group used principally
as herbicides. There are several different types. Because of its unique ability to produce lung disease, the
chemical of principal concern is paraquat. It will be
discussed in detail.

Paraquat

Paraquat is 1,1'-dimethyl-4-4'-bipyridinium chloride.
It has a structural formula of

$$\left[CH_3-N \underset{}{\bigcirc}-\underset{}{\bigcirc} N-CH_3 \right]^{2+} \quad 2Cl^-$$

The common tradenames are Gramoxone and Ortho Paraquat
or Ortho Weed and Spot Killer. The molecular formula of
the salt is $C_{12}H_{14}N_2Cl_2$. The molecular weight of the
dichloride salt is 257.2 and of the cation is 186.2. The
chemical decomposes at approximately 300°C. It is normally in a white crystalline solid state and is hygroscopic. The formulated technical grade is a dark red
solution with a rather faint ammoniacal odor. Specific
gravity is 1.24-1.26 and the vapor pressure is very low,

below 1×10^{-7} mm Hg. The chemical is principally soluble
only in water and has little to no solubility in organics.
It is available commercially as an aqueous solution and
is applied at rates of 0.25 to 1.0 pounds per acre. The
chemical does decompose under ultraviolet irradiation
with 25-50% breakdown being noted after three weeks
through photochemical decomposition. Lack of ultraviolet
radiation may allow the chemical to be retained on plant
surfaces for long periods of time. Under normal storage
conditions, the shelf life is indefinite. Following use
on crops, tolerances have been set, with the common food
residue tolerances usually in the range of 0.1-0.5 ppm
(fruits, cereals, wheat, etc.). In soil, bacteria can
decompose the paraquat metabolite methyl isonicotinic
acid to methyl amine. Further degradation to carbon
dioxide apparently can occur.

The basic toxicology of paraquat has been reviewed
by Haley (1979). In rats, the acute LD_{50} is about
21 mg/kg. The dermal LD_{50} is 80-90 mg/kg in rats. In
guinea pigs, the range is from 20-60 mg/kg for the acute
LD_{50} and in rabbits it is about 50 mg/kg. Other animals,
such as cats, hens, turkeys, cows and sheep have been
studied with similar or higher LD_{50} for the acute effect.
In monkeys, the LD_{50} has been shown to be 50-75 mg/kg.
Following acute intoxication, animals will develop symptoms or signs of vomiting, diarrhea, malaise and weight
loss. The principal acute effects appear to be damage
to the kidneys, liver and adrenal glands. Central nervous system effects will occur with very large dosages
leading to fatal convulsions.

According to the review by Haley, the literature
suggests that paraquat is neither mutagenic, carcinogenic
nor teratogenic.

Human Toxicology Experience: A considerable amount of
clinical experience has been reported in the literature
with over 100 cases of illness and/or death. The chemical is unique in the sense that there is not only an
acute toxicity syndrome but, in addition, it has the
ability to produce a delayed fibroblastic response in the
lungs. The latter is usually the principal mechanism of
death.

For industrial workers, paraquat is not considered
very dangerous. Inhalation hazard is extremely low due
to the low vapor pressure of the chemical. Nevertheless,
protective respiratory equipment should be used particularly when other atmospheric contamination might occur.

On no occasion should an applicator be allowed to walk
through drifting spray although, at least in experimental
animals, the toxic response is inversely related to
particle size, i.e. the larger the size of the inhaled
particle, the smaller the toxic lung response. Studies
by Staiff and co-workers (1975) on occupationally exposed
persons indicate that both dermal and respiratory exposure
to paraquat does not appear to present a hazard to field
applicators although absorption is easily demonstrated.
In the studies presented, a maximum of 3.5 mg/hour could
be absorbed through the dermal-respiratory route under
conditions of ordinary exposure. This would represent
0.06% of the toxic dose as compared to the LD_{50} for male
white rats. The greatest exposure occurs on the hands
and a special effort should be made to prevent skin
contact under field conditions. The particular importance of preventing splashing into the eyes or the mouth
are also noted.

Interestingly, the pulmonary manifestations of delayed
toxicity which are seen in rats and humans do not occur
in all animals. For example, no delayed fibrosis occurs
in guinea pigs. On the other hand, rats, guinea pigs,
and monkeys all have acute symptoms of intoxication.
They are: lethargy, dyspnea (from acute hemorrhagic
changes), signs of hepatic failure and acute renal failure. Microscopic examination of acutely intoxicated
animals reveals considerable paravascular cuffing with
pulmonary edema and alveolar collapse, hepatic central
lobular necrosis and renal tubular necrosis. As noted
earlier, acute necrosis of the adrenal glands has also
been demonstrated in some situations.

The toxic effects of paraquat must be divided into the
acute versus the subacute manifestations. Paraquat is a
definite irritant of both the skin and the mucous membranes. When paraquat is splashed into the eye, irritation is immediate. It may produce conjunctival damage
with one case report demonstrating temporary loss of the
tarsal conjunctiva requiring careful follow-up although
complete healing eventually occurred.

Paraquat can cause contact dermatitis, including a
severe form which has been related to edema and exuda-
tion. Repeated exposure will produce an effect upon
fingernails which is manifested by nail damage with
discoloration as a transverse white band and/or transverse ridging. This is a reversible change which ceases
after exposure. (Baran, 1974)

Following oral ingestion of paraquat, initial symptoms are burning of the mouth and throat, nausea, vomiting and diarrhea. Oral pharyngeal alterations are common and patients develop a prominant pharyngeal membrane which is highly suggestive of tonsillar-pharyngeal diphtheria. Important in distinguishing paraquat poisoning from diphtheria is the extent of the oral membrane involvement. In diphtheria, the membrane begins in the tonsils and then may spread in a confluent fashion. In paraquat poisoning, the membrane is much more extensive and involves the gums, the floor of the mouth and the tongue. Thus, the differential diagnosis includes other diseases with extensive pharyngeal pseudomembranes, such as Vincent's angina, adenoviral pharyngitis, thrush, primary herpetic tonsillitis, and a granulocytosis (Stephens, et al 1981).

The principal manifestations of acute intoxication in adults are related to the irritant and toxic effects per se. The chemical produces mucosal irritation which causes bleeding of the gastrointestinal tract. There can be abdominal pain secondary to the gastrointestinal irritation. Hepatotoxicity will produce anorexia (loss of appetite) and may even produce an obstructive jaundice. Acute renal failure may occur as a result of tubular necrosis and pulmonary edema can also occur as a direct toxic effect. Aplastic anemia has been reported in five cases (van Dijk, 1975).

Although the acute symptoms of paraquat intoxication are of concern and are dangerous, the principal problem relates to the unique delayed manifestations of this chemical's ability to produce a fibroblastic change in the lung which begins a number of days after absorption. This problem was brought to the public's attention when paraquat spraying of marijuana in Mexico became a public issue (Turner, 1978; Liddle, 1980). Interesting scientific issues were raised since previous experience seemed to demonstrate that the chemical could only produce a respiratory lesion following oral absorption. Experiments then found that it was possible to induce respiratory failure as a result of both dermal and aerosol routes of absorption (Newhouse, 1978). On the other hand, the low dosage of paraquat upon marijuana did not appear to result in significantly high enough levels to produce lung disease. Approximately 20% of all marijuana entering the country in 1976 was contaminated with paraquat but levels were low enough that most authorities did not consider it to be significant. Since crude

marijuana contains a number of chemicals which in themselves are known to be causative agents for chronic lung
disease, this situation was even more confounding.

Treatment: The principal treatment of paraquat intoxication is directed at an attempt to prevent the
absorption of the chemical into the blood with subsequent
distribution to other organs (Smith, 1974; Cavalli, 1977).
This is particularly true since there is no specific
antidote for paraquat and, therefore, every effort must
be made to prevent distribution to a sensitive organ,
such as the lung or kidney. Blood and urine samples
should be drawn and taken serially throughout the treatment. If possible, samples of gastric contents should
also be analyzed. First aid treatment for paraquat
should include removal of any of the chemical from the
skin. If swallowing has occurred, forced vomiting is
advisable.
In the Emergency Room, patients should be intubated
immediately and lavage instituted. It is important to
use some means of attempting to absorb the chemical from
the gastrointestinal tract, therefore, Fuller's earth in
a 30% w/v solution or bentonite particles in a 7.5% w/v
solution should be used. If neither of these are available, activated charcoal may be tried but it is known to
be less effective. Following lavage with 200-500 ml of
the Fuller's earth or bentonite, a saline cathartic may
be administered. The above procedure can be repeated
every two to four hours if it is suspected that further
paraquat is in the gastrointestinal tract. If absorption
has occurred, some authorities recommend hemodialysis as
a means of attempting to remove paraquat from the blood.
Forced diuresis with furosemide or with mannitol is
recommended and should be started immediately along with
intravenous fluids in order to promote renal excretion.
Because paraquat is oxidized to a more toxic peroxide
radical, oxygen is contraindicated in the treatment of
paraquat intoxication. Patients should be followed with
arterial blood gases and the only exception made to no
oxygen therapy would be if arterial blood gases become
low enough to be of concern along with the patient's
general condition. In any event, oxygen should be administered with extreme caution - even in the face of
mild respiratory distress. If absorption has occurred,
vital signs should be followed carefully and the patient
should be monitored because of the danger of acute cardiac myopathy. Renal output must be measured carefully

in case of acute renal failure. Liver function studies
should be performed routinely and serially because of the
hepatotoxic manifestations.

  Diagnostic Laboratory Studies: Patients should be
followed regularly with serial plasma paraquat concentrations. A study by Proudfoot and associates (1979)
would appear to demonstrate that those patients whose
plasma concentrations did not exceed 2.0, 0.6, 0.3, 0.16
and 0.10 mg/1 at 4, 6, 10, 16 and 24 hours respectively
are likely to have an excellent prognosis. Those patients
with higher levels at each point are much more likely to
have end-stage disease and should be treated more vigor-
ously. Plasma paraquat concentrations can be measured
by gas chromatography, radioimmunoassay or colorimetric
methods (Levitt, 1977; Jarvie, 1979).

References

Baran, R.L. (1974) Nail damage caused by weed killers
    and insecticides. Arch Dermatol 110:467.

Cavalli, R.D. and K. Fletcher (1977) An effective
    treatment for paraquat poisoning. IN: Biochemical
    Mechanisms of Paraquat Toxicity, Autor, A.P. (ed.),
    Academic Press, New York, pp 213-230.

Haley, T.J. (1979) Review of the toxicology of paraquat
    (1,1'-dimethyl-4,4'-bipyridinium chloride). Clin
    Toxicol 14:1-46.

Newhouse, M., D. McEvoy and D. Rosenthal (1978)
    Percutaneous paraquat absorption. Arch Dermatol
    114:1516-1519.

Jarvie, D.R. and M.J. Stewart (1979) The rapid
    extraction of paraquat from plasma using an ion-pair
    technique. Clin Chim Acta 94:241-251.

Levitt, T. (1977) Radioimmunoassay for paraquat.
    Lancet 2:358.

Liddle, J.A., L.L. Needham, Z.J. Rollen, R.B. Roark and
    D.D. Bayse (1980) Characterization of the contamin-
    ation of marijuana with paraquat. Bull Environ
    Contam Toxicol 24:49-53.

Popenoe, D. (1979) Effects of paraquat aerosol on
  mouse lung. Arch Pathol Lab Med 103:331-334.

Proudfoot, A.T., M.S. Stewart, T. Levitt and B. Widdop
  (1979) Paraquat poisoning: Significance of plasma-
  paraquat concentrations. Lancet 2:330-332.

Smith, L.L., A. Wright, I. Wyatt and M.S. Rose (1974)
  Effective treatment for paraquat poisoning in rats
  and its relevance to treatment of paraquat poisoning
  in man. Brit Med J 2:569-571.

Staiff, D.C., S.W. Comer, J.F. Armstrong and H.R. Wolfe
  (1975) Exposure to the herbicide paraquat.
  Bull Environ Contam Toxicol 14:334-340.

Stephens, D.S., D.H. Walker, W. Schaffner, L.G. Kaplowitz,
  H.R. Brashear, R. Roberts and W.S. Sprickard, Jr.
  (1981) Pseudodiphtheria: Prominent pharyngeal
  membrane associated with fatal paraquat ingestion.
  Ann Intern Med 94:202-204.

Turner, C.E., M.A. Elsohly, F.P. Cheng and L.M. Torres
  (1978) Marijuana and paraquat. JAMA 240:1857.

van Dijk, A., R.A.A. Maes, R.H. Drost, J.M.C. Douze and
  A.N.P. van Heyst (1975) Paraquat poisoning in man.
  Arch Toxicol 34:129-136.

4

Organophosphates

Introduction

Organophosphorus pesticide usage has increased since
the ban on the chlorinated hydrocarbons such at DDT. The
advantage of the organophosphorus pesticide group is that
they do not bioaccumulate in the environment, as some of
the chlorinated hydrocarbons do. The disadvantage is
that the chemicals are far more acutely toxic than the
chlorinated hydrocarbons. The production of these chemicals has increased at least by a third and the organophosphorus compounds are now the most widely used pesticides of all classes. An estimated 40% of all crops
have this class of pesticide applied and a substantial
contact by workers is involved. It is estimated that
approximately $4\frac{1}{2}$ million people are engaged in farm employment in the United States per year. However, at one
time or another during the year, probably as many as
8-9 million persons do some work in commercial agriculture. The differences in numbers are accounted for partly by seasonal employment with a variation in the number
of workers as the result of seasonal and geographic differences. With such large numbers of exposed workers, it
is not surprising that occupational illness is reported.
In California, a state with an active reporting system,
the organophosphates are the most common cause of herbicide or pesticide illnesses in humans. Again, in
1976, during the application of malathion water-disper-
sible powder for malaria control operations in Pakistan,
7500 field workers were exposed and poisoning occurred
in 2500 of those. Five of these individuals died. Upon

reviewing the incident, it was believed that the intox-
ications occurred partly by the failure to use elementary
precautions during the handling and spraying of the formulation - pointing up the necessity of having package
labels in the appropriate language with instructions concerning proper use and handling. The second factor involved was the suspicion that isomalathion, an impurity
found in the formulation, contributed to this incident.
This impurity is normally in very low concentrations in
technical grade malathion but is formed in larger amounts
in some of the powder formulations. In this particular
incident, using of certain inert diluents at the time of
application may have increased the level of isomalathion
after manufacture, during shipment, or during field storage. Samples of the material were found to have an isomalathion content two to five times greater than normal.
WHO (1978) recommends that the highest acceptable level
for isomalathion should be 1.8% of the normal malathion
content.

Another example of a large incident of acute organophosphate intoxication occurred in Rhodesia's Black population and was reported by Hayes and coworkers (1978).
A total of 105 patients were diagnosed as having acute
organophosphate intoxication. Of these, 44 were secondary to suicide attempts, 12 were secondary to accidental
ingestion, 11 were secondary to agricultural or industrial
contact and 38 patients did not give a positive history
of source although it was believed that symptoms were
related to the ingestion of vegetables or concoctions of
"home brew" consumed in the rural districts. Interestingly, 13 patients had a recurrence of symptoms after
discharge from the hospital and the reason for recurrence
could not be established. The author suggests, as do
others, that the re-exposure to organophosphates, even in
very small dosages, may cause a relapse of symptoms because patients may already have depleted levels of cholinesterase as the result of the severe initial exposure.
In this series, only one case of peripheral neuropathy
occurred as a long-term effect. The diagnosis was frequently based only upon clinical symptoms and signs. The
measurement of pseudocholinesterase (serum cholinesterase
by the colorometric method) was used as a screen in only
71 of the patients.

Worker Safety

The organophosphates should be stored in well-ventil-
ated areas. Workers should be advised to wear safety
glasses, long sleeved shirts or coveralls with tight
collars and cuffs. Rubber gloves are usually advisable,
as are boots. In many cases, an all-purpose cannister
should be used for protection against inhalation. Every
attempt should be made to prevent splash of the chemical
against skin surfaces.

For most workers, absorption of pesticides of this
class will occur mainly through the skin. Although
applicators are the most severely exposed workers, they
are also much more carefully protected. It is the worker
who is re-entering a field after application who may
become exposed to residues in varying concentrations
which will pass through the skin. Although some respiratory exposure may occur, the main problem still seems
to be the ability of the skin to absorb chemicals.
Absorptions through the skin have been measured with a
number of organophosphorus pesticides. Those most easily
absorbed are Guthion, Azodrin, Parathion and Malathion.
In most cases, as one increases the surface dose to the
skin, the percentage of the applied dose absorbed increases in a linear fashion. There is, however, considerable variation in the amount of absorption depending
upon the anatomic region which has been exposed (Maibach,
1971). For example, the areas of skin which absorb most
poorly are areas such as the palm and abdomen and areas
which absorb best are areas such as the antecubital
fossa, the axilla and the scrotum. Also playing a role
in the absorption problem is the total amount of excretion since it appears that certain areas will allow the
chemical to get to the blood stream more quickly and
provide for a better rate of excretion. Although the
skin is a reasonably good barrier, if there is any area
of skin damage, one can expect increased penetration up
to nearly 100%.

Many pesticide users have attempted to protect their
hands by using gloves. It has been recognized that if
there were no material on the skin before gloves were
worn, or, if the gloves are truly impermeable, this
might offer excellent protection, however, under actual
field conditions it has been demonstrated that canvas
gloves significantly increase, rather than decrease,
the penetration of organophosphates. Studies into the
nature of the weave of fabrics, as well as the effect
of various types of barrier creams, are currently in

progress. Preliminary studies would indicate that these creams may be partially effective.

Removal of organophosphorus pesticides is best accomplished by soap and water. The use of organic solvents is no more effective. Showering is also less effective than simple application of soap and water.

In the workplace, there should be no food or smoking allowed. For the workers who are going to be exposed on a regular basis to organophosphates, it is advisable to have a pre-employment cholinesterase performed for baseline and then cholinesterases repeated, possibly as often as every month, in order to determine whether or not exposure is occurring with subclinical findings. When the red blood cell or plasma cholinesterase falls to 50% of normal, workers are to be removed from the job and not return to work until cholinesterase is again at 75% of the normal value.

Accidental spills should be considered an acute medical emergency and speed is imperative. The clothing of the victim should be removed and the victim should be flushed with copious amounts of water and/or soap and water. The persons caring for the victim also should be advised to be careful of splash in this situation and should at least be wearing rubber gloves. Individuals should be transferred as soon as possible and Emergency Room personnel should be warned in advance. Persons transporting individuals with acute organophosphate exposure should be capable of performing cardiopulmonary resuscitation. With a very highly toxic chemical or with significant enough dosage, respiratory paralysis may occur leading to sudden cessation of respiration.

Spillage can be absorbed with paper towels then placed in a plastic bag and burned in an open pan or with the help of a flammable solvent in some sort of furnace. When placed in the furnace, it is probably advisable to add equal parts of sand and crushed limestone and then cover with a combustible solvent such as alcohol or benzene and finally ignite it and allow the mixture to burn thoroughly. The sand and crushed limestone can then be disposed of into a paper carton and the latter may be burned in a furnace with an afterburner and an alkali scrubber.

Re-entry Problems

The need for the development of an appropriate time interval from application to the point at which workers might be allowed to re-enter previously treated fields was recognized during the late 1960's and early 1970's. Early studies in cotton crops suggested that the residue on crops might be at variance with what was anticipated and reports of possible organophosphate intoxication syndromes began to develop in the reporting system used in California. As a result, a special committee was formed, chaired by T.H. Milby, and the results were published in 1974. In addition, the Environmental Protection Agency (1974) published a set of proposed re-entry times for a variety of chemicals using the existing guidelines. Following the report of the Special Committee on Occupational Exposure to Pesticides, regional research studies were undertaken which involved the states of Arizona, Florida, California, Oregon and Washington. The project was terminated in 1979. The major objectives were the following:

1. To develop information to be used in establishing safe worker re-entry intervals for pesticide treated crops. This was performed by studies of dislodgeable and soil-dust residues which established levels which were occurring on the crops of interest.

2. To determine principles governing the factors which affect safe re-entry intervals. Studies were performed on the chemical and physical factors important to re-entry worker exposure to possibly hazardous pesticide residues.

3. To encourage and corroborate with clinical studies, the verification of these principles. The latter objective was not finished because of resistence to human subject experimental studies.

Presently, the allowable re-entry time varies from state to state. Studies indicate that dislodgeable residues are an important determining factor and that the amounts of dislodgeable residues vary with climate

and with crop. For example, in California where regulations for re-entry are sometimes tighter than the federal regulations, the 1976 Administrative Code allows for
a six day re-entry time for grape orchards versus a 21
day re-entry time for peach orchards for the same organophosphate, methylparathion. A number of similar variations also exist in the federal regulations.

Although there has been no verification of fatal cases
of poisoning from organophosphate residues related to re-
entry, there have been numerous non-fatal cases of intoxication in a variety of crops and in a number of geographic areas. Principally, these have occurred in
California with another high suspect area initially
being in the South, particularly in Florida. There is a
disproportionate distribution of recognized poisoning
incidents occurring in California compared to the rest
of the nation. The exact mechanism for this dispropor-
tion remains unknown. At one time, it was felt to be
accounted for by the differences in temperature and
climate in California as compared for example to Florida,
however, studies have not substantiated this hypothesis.

The problem of worker safety re-entry intervals has
also been addressed in Europe and a publication by
Derache (1977) is a thorough review of the toxicity of
the commonly used organophosphates as well as the dose-
response relationships which have been used to develop
appropriate re-entry intervals.

The recognition of an acute intoxication syndrome from
organophosphates such as might occur from an accidental
spill or from suicidal intent is a relatively simple
process. On the other hand, recognition of subtle effects which might occur from long-term exposure is considerably more difficult.

The occupationally exposed worker is at risk for
organophosphate intoxication. While it is clear that
workers can be exposed on a repeated basis without any
symptoms or signs, it is also true, that unless very
careful protective measures are taken during such times
of exposure, particularly for such people as formulators
or mixers, a gradual depression of cholinesterase may
occur without the development of frank symptoms. Because
of the nature of this depression, workers should be
monitored on a routine basis with cholinesterase levels
and removed from the job when a depression of 50% from
the baseline level has occurred. It has been shown that
with appropriate working conditions which are designed
for preventing absorption, workers can work safely with
these chemicals without depression of cholinesterase and

certainly without symptoms or signs of intoxication. In addition to formulators and applicators of the organo-phosphate pesticides, workers involved in harvesting crops must adhere carefully to re-entry standards which have been set in order to prevent the asymptomatic de-pression of cholinesterase and the possibility of the development of an insidious, but low level, chronic in-toxication syndrome (Knaak, 1978; Owens, 1978; Wolfe, 1978).

Acute Organophosphate Intoxication

Namba, et al (1971) were the first to thoroughly review the organophosphorus pesticide compounds with respect to clinical manifestations and recommendations for treatment. In addition, this review was oriented toward basic physiology and biochemistry of the chemicals and, in discussing the clinical changes, they summarized the effect of cholinesterase depression by characterizing the effects as being either 1) muscarinic, 2) nicotinic, or 3) central nervous system effects. The muscarinic effects of cholinesterase depression were related to actions on the bronchi and stimulation of the salivary, lacrimal and sweat glands, etc., resulting in secondary signs of pulmonary edema, tearing and sweating. The nicotinic effects were the secondary changes noted in the skeletal-motor system and also in the sympathetic nervous system which lead to findings of fasciculation, muscle weakness, tachycardia and diarrhea. The central nervous system effects were related entirely to giddiness, anxiety, emotional lability, ataxia, confusion, and severe central nervous system depression. Namba felt that the neurological problems were primarily a peripher-al neuropathy involving a number of different types of nerves and discounted the possibility of any cause-effect relationship upon the central nervous system which might be of a chronic nature. Indeed, he felt that such changes were mainly of an "emotional origin".

The first review of the neurological manifestations of organophorphorus insecticide poisoning which recog-nized central nervous system effects as a clinical man-ifestation was then published by Wadia and co-workers (1974). In a review of the neurological findings in 200 consecutive cases of suicidal ingestion of organo-phosphosphorus insecticides, these investigators found definite evidence of central nervous system disease.

They classified the spectrum of neurological changes into two types. The type 1 signs, those usually present on admission, were chiefly from the immediate effect of peripheral cholinesterase depression and caused impaired consciousness and pyramidal tract signs but responded to atropine. Type 2 signs were related to complaints which appeared later – while the patients were on atropine treatment. The most common signs noted were proximal limb weakness, areflexia and cranial nerve palsy. Of 36 cases classified as type 2 paralysis, 15 died from respiratory paralysis after variable periods from the onset and 21 recovered with no residual neurological deficits described. Wadia emphasized that a correlation of delayed neurological deficits with cholinesterase depression was poor. Indeed, he felt that there was no correlation and that the delayed clinical signs were the result of changes in the spinal cord at the anterior horn cells.

Early studies, prior to the review by Wadia, implicated several organophosphates capable of producing delayed central nervous system signs, namely ipafox and leptophos. A number of clinical studies have now appeared which strongly suggest that central nervous system involvement may be manifested as changes only in the cranial nerves. In particular, optic neuropathy, manifested mainly as severe myopia in school children, has been ascribed to organophosphates by a number of Japanese workers (Tamura, 1978; Ishikawa, 1978; Uchida, 1974). In an epidemiological study of 324 children and 255 adults, Ishikawa noted ocular signs which included diminished visual acuity, narrowing of the peripheral visual field and/or central scotomata, myopia and astigmatism. These were all ascribed to organophosphate pesticides although exact cause and effect for all signs may be difficult to completely prove. In these studies, laboratory tests did demonstrate organophosphate pesticide levels in blood and urine with reduction in cholinesterase activity and liver function abnormalities. In addition, studies by the same author on beagles who were given ethylthiometon at varying dosages for two years also demonstrated visual changes. Involvement of the eighth cranial nerve has been implicated in a case report of acute bilateral permanent sensorineural hearing loss which occurred following poisoning from combined exposure to an aerosol of malathion and methoxychlor (Harrell, 1978). Although not clearly cause and effect, a case of Guillain-Barré syndrome has also been reported by Fisher

(1977) which occurred following dermal absorption of
merphos. In this case cholinesterase levels were not
performed and the acute Guillain-Barre occurred only a
matter of hours after exposure. Thus the typical picture
of delayed neurological disease was not present (Harrell,
1978).

Chronic Organophosphate Intoxication

Following recovery from an episode of organophosphate
intoxication in which the cholinesterase is depressed
and secondary manifestations of neurological signs have
occurred, the principal concern is the development of a
delayed syndrome which is neuromuscular and/or neuropsychiatric in nature. Prior to the development of
organophosphorus compounds as insecticides, experience
with a neurotoxic organophosphate compound, triortho-
cresyl phosphate (TOCP), occurred. From this episode,
considerable clinical experience developed. The report
of this widespread poisoning epidemic which occurred in
1930 has been reviewed by Morgan and Penovich (1978).
Basically, the episode involved an illegal alcoholic
beverage, called Jamaica ginger extract or "jake", which
contained a solvent used as an ingredient in varnish.
The disease was widespread in the South where local laws
prohibited legal alcohol. Initially, the syndrome was
felt to be a peripheral neuritis however follow-up of
some of these cases has demonstrated that the central
nervous system was clearly involved and that the actual
residual effect was an upper motor neuron lesion. Apparently the discrepancy was due to the initial syndrome
being a lower motor neuron type with areflexia and flac-
cidity. With time, in some patients, the peripheral
nerve manifestation disappeared and the supervening
spinal cord changes then developed.
One of the earliest studies alluding to the possible
chronic neurological effects from insecticides was performed by Davignon and co-workers (1965). This study
examined 441 workers who used insecticides in their
occupation, a group of 170 persons living in the same
environment and a group of 162 other persons having no
contact whatsoever with insecticides. Objective findings
of miosis, decreased reflexes, tremors and disturbances
of equilibrium were found. The findings were correlated
not only with contacts versus controls but the incidence
of neurological abnormalities increased with duration of

exposure, i.e. there was a time related correlation.
A mild leukopenia was also noted among these workers.
The study was not definitive because workers used a
wide variety of insecticides including chlorinated hydrocarbons, carbamates, amines, organic material, inorganic
insecticides and others. Trichlorphon delayed neuropathy
has been reported by Ikuta (1973). In this case, an 81
year old farmer attempted suicide by swallowing 65 ml of
50% trichlorphon. Following the acute episode of intoxication, he developed a delayed neurological syndrome
consisting of ataxia, muscular atrophy, hyporeflexia
and hypoesthesia beginning on the 27th day after ingestion. A report by Hierons and Johnson (1978) described
a case of delayed neuropathy secondary to trichlorphon
(also known as chlorphos and marketed as Dipterex).
Symptoms of the neuropathy did not begin until eight
days after the acute poisoning and progressed for about
two months. The weakness was predominantly distal,
which seems to be a rather characteristic finding.
Since trichlorphon is metabolized to dichlorvos, the
authors suggest that the latter may have been the cause
of the delayed neuropathy. A major point made was that
perhaps neurotoxicity screening should be expanded in
the pre-marketing phase. Gadoth and Fisher (1978) report
an interesting case of acute malathion intoxication
secondary to ingestion of 150 ml of a commercial preparation of malathion and 50% xylene in an attempt to
commit suicide. About two days after recovery from the
acute illness, the patient proceeded to develop ptosis,
external ophthalmoplegia, proximal muscle weakness and
areflexia. This patient was treated with both atropine
and obidoxime (Toxogonin). In spite of the latter treatment, she developed the late paralytic signs, or type 2
as described by Wadia, and this was contrary to previous
experience. In Israel, where the use of 2-PAM or Toxogonin is routine in all cases of organophosphorus poisoning, late-onset paralysis was not noticed among 198
reported cases. A possible mechanism proposed is that
in some patients there is a late release of previously
inactivated cholinesterase inhibitor which acts specifically on the "nicotinic" receptors and thereby causes a
secondary, or delayed, neuropathy. Since metabolic
studies have never been performed on patients of this
sort, it is also conceivable that some type of storage,
either of parent compound or some breakdown product,
occurs and then is released in a delayed fashion to
reproduce some of the syndrome.

Neurological complaints are not to be expected in cases of either routine occupational exposure or even in all cases of suicidal intent. Kraus and co-workers (1977) report the physiologic response of 21 male agricultural workers exposed to Guthion residues in which medical examination before and after exposure revealed an absence of clinical signs of organophosphate intoxication although there was a mild decrease in the cholinesterase values noted after exposure. The authors do suggest that there may also have been some mild hyporeflexia which occurred. A study by Jusic (1978) of two patients who attempted suicide via the ingestion of malathion did not demonstrate any evidence of neurological disease after the recovery, including normal electromyographic examination. Studies in Sweden by Stalberg and co-workers (1978) have also been performed and did not demonstrate any evidence of changes in neuromuscular function after occupational exposure to organophosphorus insecticides. An investigation of agricultural workers primarily exposed to organophosphate insecticides in which a standardized method of measuring Achilles reflex was used demonstrated a significant decrease in reflex force of the high organophosphate users versus a control population but this is not a delayed effect. No changes in EMG spike potential were noted in these workers nor were changes in nerve conduction velocity (Rayner, 1972). An interesting study by Fenichel and co-workers (1972) used paraoxon, the toxic breakdown product of parathion. Rats administered 0.25 mg/kg of paraoxon demonstrated a histological picture of myopathy with a focal necrosis followed by fibronecrosis and phagocytosis.

Behavior Changes

A questionable side effect, but one which is both intriguing and poorly understood, is the possibility of psychiatric changes occurring with exposure to some organophosphates. In a very thorough review on the effect of organophosphate poisoning in occupational workers in California, Tabershaw (1966) notes the relative absence of neuropsychiatric sequelae following acute intoxication. That is, he felt the number of individuals who had severe manifestations such as anxiety, depression or personality changes was not striking and no psychoses were reported in any of 114 cases which he examined. On the other hand, he did note that during periods of recurrent exposure, after an acute episode of intoxication,

many individuals commented upon irritability, insomnia
and inability to concentrate and then seemed to recover
completely after the new exposure ceased. This intolerance to a very slight contact with organophosphate
insecticides was fairly common to individuals after acute
poisoning. Tabershaw concludes that "this intolerance,
psychogenic or not, appears to be a real after effect".
It was early noted that low toxicity organophosphates
such as malathion could be given to rats without any
changes in cholinesterase levels but with the production
of anesthesia (Vandekar 1957). Studies by Durham, Wolfe
and Quinby (1965) on occupationally exposed workers
indicate that mental alertness is decreased but only in
those cases where there are other absolute signs and
symptoms of intoxication. Similarly, a neurobehavioral
study by Rodnitzky, Levin and Mick (1975) was performed
with exposed workers being tested for abnormalities in
memory, signal processing, vigilance, language and proprioceptive feedback performance. They concluded that
the performance of exposed workers was not deficient in
any of the five measures assessed. A resistance to the
effects of DFP was noted in a study by Rowntree, Nevin
and Wilson (1950) in which the administration of DFP
caused fewer effects in the schizophrenic patients than
in controls with manic depressive patients being somewhat
intermediary. Lethargy appeared to be a significant side
effect in this investigation. A report by Sidell (1974)
is of interest. In this report, four patients were
accidently exposed tc Sarin and one was similarly exposed
to Soman. The two with the most severe intoxication had
psychiatric sequelae which persisted for many weeks.
Interestingly, the use of scopolamine (and a blind control) ameliorated the mental condition in one patient
rather than the expected opposite effect. Recovery of
the pupils' ability to dilate was delayed and is a prob-
able explanation for chronic complaints of difficulty
focusing after acute intoxication. A report by Dille
and Smith (1964) of two cases of intoxication indicates
that the primary symptoms were anxiety, uneasiness and
depression in one case and ataxia, anxiety, emotional
lability and inability to perform familiar tasks in the
second case.

   Electroencephalographic changes will also occur during
some kinds of acute human organophosphate intoxication.
Such studies are reported by Brown (1971) and by Wood
and co-workers (1971). In one instance, the electroencephalographic changes persisted for two years following the episode of intoxication. Similarly, prolonged

and definitive changes occurred in an acute episode of
intoxication secondary to Sarin (Dille and Smith, 1964).
Finally, Duffy and co-workers (1979) have examined elec-
troencephalograms on a number of workers exposed to Sarin
and indicated a difference between the EEG's of workers
versus those of control groups. The differences included
increased beta activity, increased delta and theta slow-
ing, decreased alpha activity and increased amounts of
rapid eye movement (REM) sleep.

Mechanisms of Delayed Neurotoxicity

The development of a delayed neuropathy in association
with organophosphates is a distinctly different clinical
syndrome than the acute neurotoxicity seen as a manifestation of cholinesterase inhibition at the peripheral
neuromuscular junction. The clinical syndrome of delayed
neuropathy is not seen for up to 14 days after the acute
syndrome and may even be seen when the patient becomes
clinically "well" as the result of atropine therapy in
the initial stages of intoxication. At the onset of the
delayed syndrome, weakness and ataxia will predominate,
usually developing first in the lower limbs and then
typically progressing through a paralysis which may even
affect the upper limbs. In this sense, the syndrome can
mimic a Guillain-Barré, however, a distinction should be
made simply by the history of significant exposure.
The delayed neuropathy syndrome was perhaps first
associated with a prospective organophosphate pesticide,
Mipafox, when workers engaged in the laboratory production of this chemical developed a delayed neurotoxic
effect. Prior to this, it was thought that the delayed
effect of organophosphates in general was specific to
the triaryl phosphates, however, the association with
Mipafox demonstrated that alkyl phosphoryl esters could
also play a role. Today, it is known that a number of
different agents or their metabolic products may contribute in the development of delayed neuropathy. Indeed,
a method has been developed whereby organophosphates may
be screened prior to manufacture and may be rated according to the degree of neurotoxicity. This is discussed in
a review by Johnson (1975), one of the key workers in
this field.
In a series of investigations, Johnson demonstrated
what he first thought to be a "neurotoxic protein" found
in the central nervous system. His later studies showed

that, in fact, an esterase was present rather than a
protein and that when 80% or more of this neurotoxic
esterase was inhibited, the delayed neurotoxic effect
would become a clinical syndrome. It now appears that
there are two classes of inhibitors, both of which com-
bine covalently to the active site of the neurotoxic
esterase; however, the chemical classes falling into the
phosphates, the phosporamidates and the phosphonates are
neurotoxic while those in the chemical classes of sulfo-
nates, the phosphinates and the carbamates are non-neuro-
toxic or may even be protective. The inhibition of the
neurotoxic esterase is believed to occur through a process often referred to as "aging" since it is time-depen-
dent. This fact accounts for the need to treat clinical
organophosphate intoxication rapidly so the delayed
neurotoxic phenomenon from the "aging" phenomenon does
not occur.

Histologically, delayed neurotoxicity was initially
referred to as a "demyelinating disease". This mistaken
conclusion was drawn from examination of peripheral
lesions which demonstrated a loss of the myelin sheath
surrounding the long nerve axons. Later work has clearly
demonstrated that demyelinization is not the primary
process and that demyelinating disease is not an appropriate classification. Rather, both light and electron
microscopic studies in a variety of species show that the
actual lesion is the degeneration of the axon itself.
Such degeneration occurs both in the brain and in the
peripheral nerves.

Treatment of Organophosphate Intoxication

Review of the Clinical Syndrome

Symptoms can be expected to develop within minutes or
up to approximately 12 hours following exposure to an
organophosphate. Although the acute syndrome is divided
into the muscarinic and nicotinic phases, the two obviously cross and it is therefore best to address the entire
picture which is presented.

Early complaints may simply be fatigue, headache, some
mild vertigo, weakness and loss of concentration. As
intoxication becomes more severe, myosis becomes a prominent sign, tremor or muscle fasciculations develop,
nausea develops with associated abdominal cramps and
vomiting and eventually diarrhea develops. Excessive

sweating, tearing and salivation are observed along with
bradycardia. Finally, muscular paralysis may develop
leading to sudden respiratory arrest or depression.
Central nervous system signs develop with mental confusion, toxic psychosis, coma or convulsions.

Although the syndrome can be recognized clinically,
confirmation must be made through the use of a cholinesterase level, preferably RBC or plasma although
serum cholinesterase is usually the only test available
at most hospitals and can advantageously be quickly
performed.

Measurement of Cholinesterase Activity

Cholinesterase enzyme levels are very selective and
sensitive measurements of organophosphate intoxication.
A number of methods of measurement exist. All methods
suffer certain problems of reliability and precision.
It also must be remembered that there are two enzymes
which are measured in whole blood. One is the enzyme
attached to the red blood cell. This is the isoenzyme
which is of specific concern in organophosphate intoxication and is the enzyme responsible for inactivating
cholinesterase at the muscle endplate. The other isoenzyme is carried in the plasma and is usually referred
to as pseudocholinesterase. The latter enzyme apparently
is responsible for the inactivation of different drugs,
but not the organophosphates. Its function seems mainly
related to the pharmakokinetics of alkaloids. The plasma
cholinesterase is a genetically carried trait. It is
occasionally missing, at an estimated rate of 3/1,000
population. In these instances, individuals who are
exposed to chemicals such as scopolamine are faced with
the possibility of sudden respiratory arrest, a situation
which is occasionally seen during surgery. The safety of
workers who have a pseudocholinesterase deficiency is
uncertain. Since it is an isoenzyme, it would seem that
a low plasma cholinesterase might not be very significant
to the worker's safety; however, it has always been
deemed advisable to not expose these workers to organophosphates. Therefore, those people who are going to
have regular exposure to the organophosphates, particularly heavy exposure as might be seen in applicators, are
advised to routinely have an RBC and plasma cholinesterase
performed prior to the start of employment. The principal
methods of measuring RBC cholinesterase are those of

Michel (1949) and the pH-stat method of Nabb and
Whitfield (1967). The Michel method measures change
in pH due to the liberation of acetic acid by the enzymatic cleavage of acetocholine over a specific period of
time. The pH is allowed to change to a specific range,
the amount of change being linear with the amount of
acetic acid produced. The results are then expressed in
changes of acidity per hour as ΔpH/hour units.

In the pH-stat method, the pH of the reaction mixture
is constantly monitored with the pH meter which in turn
controls an automatic titrator. The acetic acid liber-
ated by the enzymatic cleavage of the substrate is neu-
tralized with the standardized solution of NaOH and
thereby the pH is maintained at a constant value. The
cholinesterase activity is measured in units called micro
Moles ACh/min/ml.

Unfortunately, most hospitals do not have the equipment to perform either a Michel or a pH-stat method and
the cholinesterases are routinely sent to specialized
laboratories. On the other hand, almost all hospitals
are capable of performing a pseudocholinesterase measurement on serum which is usually performed by colorometric method. A variety of methods exist for the performance of this test. The pseudocholinesterase is
reliable for screening of suspected intoxication but is
not, in itself, confirmatory and is not a good test for
measuring long-term follow-up of workers. Because of
the quick turn-around time, it is used routinely in
emergency situations, however, confirmation still requires the use of a more sophisticated method which
measures cholinesterase level in the red blood cells.

In addition to the complexity and cost of equipment,
there are other concerns with all cholinesterase measurements, particularly, the need to freeze samples immediately after drawing and to immediately perform the
measurement after thawing. The longer the material is
allowed to stand, the more significant are the errors
which can occur with any method.

Results of analysis of cholinesterase tests by Yager,
et al (1976) point out the necessity of careful laboratory control on a day to day basis in the determination
of the cholinesterase test. Indeed, if such quality
control does not occur, the variation in a single individual's values on two consecutive days would have to
differ about 30% for RBC activity and 40% for plasma in
order to conclude that a true difference existed at the
95% confidence level. Even given the quality control

on a day to day basis, this would still only reduce the necessary variance to 15% and 25% for red cells and plasma respectively. Confirmation of such variability in and between laboratories was confirmed by Burkart, et al (1977) comparing two commercial laboratories and five commercially available cholinesterase methods.

One frequently unrecognized mechanism for fall in plasma cholinesterase activity is pregnancy. Studies on healthy women in the first trimester of pregnancy demonstrated that cholinesterase will fall. No mechanism has been given for this phenomenon, however, this fact should be considered in an unexplained cholinesterase drop (Howard, et al, 1978).

Medical Treatment

Organophosphate exposure and possible intoxication are to be considered an acute emergency. Treatment should be directed, simultaneously, at first aid as well as the specific therapy. It is desirous to both attempt the prevention of further absorption and also to immed-iately start the specific therapy in order to prevent the development of a full-blown acute intoxication syn-drome and also to prevent the potential development of the delayed neuropathy which is seen with certain organo-phosphates.

First aid is not significantly different from any other water soluble toxin. Contaminated clothes should be immediately removed and the skin should be washed with soap and water. If the patient is awake and alert, Syrup of Ipecac may be used to induce vomiting, however, if there is any impairment of consciousness, the patient should be intubated and aspiration and lavage performed using isotonic saline or 5% sodium bicarbonate. Although water soluble, the chemical may be utilized in a petro-leum vehicle and caution must be undertaken to prevent the development of aspiration into the lungs. Following aspiration and removal of the gastric contents (for later analysis), activated charcoal may be instilled into the stomach along with a salt cathartic.

Specific therapy should be instituted immediately. The drug of choice is atropine sulfate which is prefer-ably given intravenously, or intramuscularly. It is important to give atropine in large dosages, i.e. 2-4 mg every 15 minutes. This should be continued until atro-pinization occurs or until there is complete reversal of

the symptoms and signs. Atropinization would be manifested by dryness of the skin and mouth, dilated pupils,
a flushing of the skin, a tachycardia of about 140/min
and diminished bowel sounds. Following atropinization
or reversal of symptoms, atropine should be continued
intravenously while the patient is watched. Excessive
atropinization may include, particularly, the development
of a fever and delirium occurring after the patient has
initially improved.

The pralidoxime, 2-PAM (Protopam by Ayerst), is also
considered a drug of choice for moderate and severe
poisoning by organophosphates. Some toxicologists believe that a pralidoxime should be used in all cases of
organophosphate intoxication. This is a matter of controversy. The purpose behind treating all patients
would be to attempt prevention of the "aging" process
with a cholinesterase inhibiting chemical. On the other
hand, the danger of pralidoxime is that the drug can,
by itself, produce a syndrome which is similar to that
of organophosphate intoxication and, therefore, will
confuse the clinical picture. Certainly the chemical
should be given in all cases of severe intoxication
with advanced central nervous system signs. Unless
there is quick reversal with atropine, it should also
be given in all moderate cases. The dosage should be
administered according to the package insert, which is
to give approximately 1.0 gram intravenously in saline
over a 30-60 minute period. In children, the dosage
should be 20-40 mg/kg. The dose may be repeated every
three to eight hours.

Certain drugs are contraindicated with suspected
organophosphate intoxication. They are morphine, aminophylline, the phenothiazine classes and reserpine.
Also, adrenergic amines should be given only if there
is a specific indication - again because of interference
with the treatment regimen. With severe central nervous
system signs such as convulsions, diazapam or related
compounds may be utilized.

Patients should be carefully monitored in the early
stages, including both ECG's and EEG's. Return to work
should be allowed only after cholinesterase is again
normal.

Human Exposure Studies - Summary of the Literature

With a number of different organophosphates, humans
have either voluntarily ingested these compounds or

studies on acutely ill patients have been done. These
studies accurately allowed for determination of dose.
This material has been summarized by the Working Group
headed by Derache (1977) and is briefly stated below.

Azinphos-Methyl: Men have swallowed 16 mg azinphosmethyl daily for 30 days. Excretion of anthranilic
acid occurred as a measure of exposure. The blood cholinesterase activity was unchanged during treatment at
this dosage.

Bromphos: Workers exposed to bromphos for two years
showed no change in RBC cholinesterase levels in one
study. In another study, eight volunteers were employed
spraying bromphos for 6.5 hours/day for 14 days. There
was no evidence of clinical illness although plasma
cholinesterase activity was slightly decreased, at a
maximum of 25% and returned to normal within one month.

Chlorfenvinphos: Eleven adult workers were exposed
for four hours on the skin of the forearm to between
five and 10 mg/kg of chlorfenvinphos. The chemical was
identified in the blood and the dosage produced a reduction in plasma cholinesterase.

Dichlorvos: Adult men exposed to dichlorvos via
atmospheric concentrations have shown conflicting results. In one study, concentrations of 6.9 mcg/1 of air
showed no reduction of cholinesterase activity. In
another study, a single exposure of eight hours at concentrations varying between 0.9 and 3.5 mcg/1 produced
very slight inhibition of plasma cholinesterase. In
workers exposed for periods of 8-10½ hours, four nights
a week for 11 straight weeks, and at atmospheric concentrations averaging 0.24 mcg/1, no change in cholinesterase was seen. A dose of 1 mg/man/day produced a
slight reduction in plasma cholinesterase. Men have
inhaled air containing dichlorvos in concentrations of
52 mg/m^3 for 62 minutes and 13 mg/m^3 for 240 minutes
with no evidence of clinical illness and only a slight
decrease in plasma cholinesterase activity. Studies of
air concentrations resulting from dichlorvos strips
which were hung in rooms and allowed for maximum concentrations of 0.1-0.2 mg/m^3 have been performed for
exposure of 28 days. During this type of exposure, no
clinical symptoms developed in subjects living in these
homes and plasma and RBC cholinesterase activities did
not change.

Ingestion of dichlorvos at a dose of 5 mg/day for a total of 20 days has been studied in men with a drop in plasma cholinesterase activity of up to 75% of the initial value. No clinical symptoms were produced and the administration did not influence the RBC cholinesterase activity. Similarly, studies have been performed in hospitalized patients in which concentrations of up to 0.28 mg/m^3 for dichlorvos for periods of three to seven days have occurred. Reduction in plasma cholinesterase activity of between 35 and 70% occurred without the expected reduction in RBC cholinesterase activity. Similarly, rooms where dichlorvos strips were hung in the delivery areas were studied where concentrations of 0.1 mg/m^3 were reached. Babies, sick children, and female patients in labor or postpartum were exposed to these vapors and also showed an inhibition of plasma cholinesterase activity without inhibition of RBC cholinesterase. Healthy neonates were exposed for 18 hours per day for five days in an atmosphere of 0.15 mg/m^3 and no drop in RBC cholinesterase activity was observed.

Demeton: Five subjects received technical demeton for 30 days at a dose of approximately 4 mg/day. During administration, no cholinesterase changes or clinical symptoms developed.

Diazinon: Subjects have received doses of 0-5 mg/kg diazinon daily for five days with a marked reduction of cholinesterase activity in the plasma but not in the erythrocytes. In another test, four individuals received the same dose for a total of 32 days without any change in either plasma or RBC cholinesterase. Finally, three adults received a daily dose of 0.05 mg/kg diazinon for five days and after an interruption of 23 days, the subjects then received the same dose for another five days; it was observed that plasma cholinesterase was decreased by 65%. Administration to adults at a dose of 0.25 mg/kg for 43 days led to a drop of plasma cholinesterase but not RBC cholinesterase.

Dimethoate: Two subjects ingested 2.5 mg of dimethoate, or 0.04 mg/kg body weight per day for over four weeks without any clinical effects or changes in cholinesterase activity. Daily doses of 5, 15, 30, 45 and 60 mg of dimethoate were administered to volunteers for periods of 14-57 days. At concentrations of 5 and 15 mg/day no effect on cholinesterase was seen but effects were noticed at dosages of 30 mg or higher.

Fenchlorfos: Male volunteers ingested an average of 11.9 mg/kg/day which led to development of symptoms as well as reduction of plasma and RBC cholinesterase.

Fenitrothion: Single oral doses of between 2.5 and 20 mg of fenitrothion have been given, corresponding to 0.042-0.33 mg/kg body weight. The urine excretion was followed by a metabolite, 3-methyl-4-nitrophenol, and was almost complete within 24 hours with an excretion peak occurring at 12 hours. Plasma cholinesterase did not decline nor were the subjects made ill.

Malathion: Male volunteers ingested 8 mg of malathion daily for 32 days without symptoms and without changes in cholinesterase. No effects were observed in a group who ingested 16 mg/day, however, cholinesterase activity did occur in groups who ingested 24 mg/day for 56 days.

Mevinphos: Volunteers ingested mevinphos at dosages of 1, 1.5, 2 and 12.5 mg/man/day for one month. Approximately a 20% reduction of RBC cholinesterase activity occurred at dosages of 1.5 and 2 mg/man/day with no significant change in plasma cholinesterase at these dose levels.

Methidathion: One subject received 0.04 mg/kg/day for 17 days and 0.08 mg/kg/day for 27 days with no effects seen on cholinesterase. Two groups of eight men received dosages of 0.04 and 0.11 mg/kg body weight per day for six weeks without any observed effects.

Parathion: Five subjects received parathion at 3 mg/day for 28 days, 4.5 mg/day for 28 days and 6 mg/day for 43 days. At the two lower dosages, plasma and RBC cholinesterase levels were not changed and at the highest dose, only a 10-15% inhibition of cholinesterase occurred. Another group was given dosages of up to 7.2 mg/day with the largest dose leading to a plasma and RBC cholinesterase decrease of 63 and 84% respectively. Over three weeks, men and women received a diet containing up to 0.05 mg parathion/kg body weight without any significant effects on cholinesterase. In subjects receiving 7 mg/day of methyl-parathion for 27 days, a reduction of approximately 15% in plasma cholinesterase was observed.

Biochemistry of Common Organophosphates

A number of good references to the complete biochemistry and mechanisms of action of organophosphates exist.
The following section is meant only to discuss the biochemistry, environmental fate and basic toxicology of
the more commonly used organophosphates in the Pacific
Northwest. Worker protection, clinical disease and
treatment are as discussed earlier.

Phosphamidon

Phosphamidon, marketed under the name Dimecron, chemically is a chloro-diethylcarbamoyl-dimethyl phosphate.
The chemical structure is as follows:

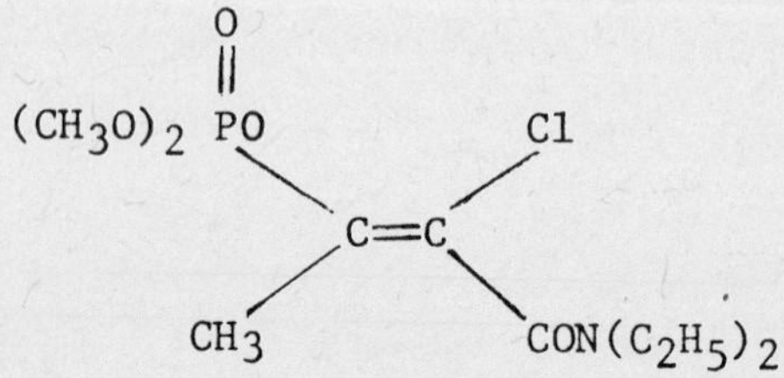

$$(CH_3O)_2 \; PO \quad\quad Cl$$

$$C{=}C$$

$$CH_3 \quad\quad CON(C_2H_5)_2$$

cis (B)-phosphamidon

It is manufactured from the chlorination of diethyl-
acetoacetamide with sulfuryl chloride and then synthesized
by Perkow reaction with a trimethyl phosphite. The
technical product is a mixture of cis and trans isomers
in the proportion 73:27. In the process of synthesis,
the product is contaminated with small quantities of
monochloro and trichloro derivatives, which, although
they are more toxic, are also more rapidly biodegradable.
    The chemical is a liquid with a boiling point of 150°C.
It is miscible with water and most organic solvents and is
only slightly soluble in alkanes. The chemical is used
for sucking pests and in the Pacific Northwest is particularly used in the treatment of apples.

Phosalone

Phosalone, also registered as Zolone and chemically
called diethyl phosphorothiolothionate has the following
chemical structure:

$$(C_2H_5O)_2P\overset{\displaystyle S}{\overset{\|}{}}-S-CH_2-N$$

The chemical is manufactured by the condensation of a chlorobenzoxazolone with a phosphorodithioate. It is a colorless crystal in liquid with a slight garlic odor. The melting point is 47°C. It is soluble in most organic solvents except the aliphatic hydrocarbons and it is readily hydrolyzed by alkalies to form 6-chlorobenzoxazolone, formaldehyde, and diethyl phosphorodithioate. The chemical is used as a broad spectrum insecticide and acaricide and is principally used for control of caterpillers, aphids and active stages of mites. The acute oral LD_{50} for male rats is 120 mg/kg.

Di-syston

The chemical formula of di-syston is as follows:

$$\begin{array}{c} C_2H_5O \\ {}\diagdown \\ C_2H_5O \diagup {} \end{array}\!\!\overset{\displaystyle S}{\overset{\|}{P}}-S-CH_2-CH_2-SC_2H_5$$

The chemical is an insecticide particularly used on wheat crops and potatoes.

Chemical Properties: It is a colorless liquid with a boiling point of 113°C. Water solubility is 25 ppm and it is soluble in most organic solvents. The molecular weight is 258.41 and the specific gravity is 1.144.

Experimental Toxicity: The chemical is toxic to mammals with oral LD_{50} in male and female rats at 12.5 and 2.5 mg/kg respectively. The oral LD_{50} in birds is 3.2 mg/kg. The chemical can react with alkylating agents leading to a secondary sulfonium compound which has strong anticholinesterase activity and high mammalian toxicity but has no insecticidal activity.

TEPP

TEPP, also called tetraethyl pyrophosphate, is a commonly used insecticide on hops. The chemical structure is as follows:

$$C_2H_5O \underset{C_2H_5O}{\overset{O}{\underset{\|}{P}}} - O - \underset{OC_2H_5}{\overset{O}{\underset{\|}{P}}} OC_2H_5$$

Chemical Properties: TEPP has a molecular weight of 290.19. The specific gravity is 1.120. The boiling point is 135-138°C. It is normally a colorless liquid and is soluble in water, alcohol, benzene and acetone. It has hygroscopic properties.

Experimental Toxicity: The oral LD_{50} in rats is 500 mcg/kg. The skin LD_{50} in rats is 20 mg/kg. The intraperitoneal LD_{50} in rats is 850 mcg/kg. In rabbits, the skin LD_{50} is 850 mg/kg. Birds are particularly susceptible with an oral LD_{50} of 1 mg/kg.

Manufacture: TEPP is synthesized by the reaction of diethyl phosphite with diethyl phosphorochloridate followed by subsequent oxidation. Preparations of TEPP are frequently contaminated with triethyl phosphate. They are easily analyzed separately with mass spectrometry. The chemical is principally degraded by hydrolysis.

Demeton (Systox)

Demeton is commonly used by its synonym of Systox. It has the chemical structure of:

$$CH_3CHO \underset{CH_3CH_2O}{\overset{S}{P}} OCH_2CH_2SCH_2CH_3 \quad + \quad CH_3CHO \underset{CH_3CHO}{\overset{S}{P}} SCH_2CH_2OCH_2CH_3$$

Chemical Properties: Demeton has a molecular weight of 258.34 and a boiling point of 134°C. It is commonly a mixture of Demeton-O and Demeton-S (Isosystox). It is normally a colorless liquid at room temperature. Solubility in water is 60 ppm and it is highly soluble in most

organic solvents including aliphatic hydrocarbons. The
chemical is metabolized to a sulfoxide isomer and then
further metabolized to a sulfone.

Experimental Toxicity: It is highly toxic in animals.
In rats the oral LD_{50} is 1.7 mg/kg. The skin LD_{50} in
rats is 200 mg/kg and the intraperitoneal LD_{50} in rats
is 3 mg/kg. The chemical is teratogenic in a number of
animals. The teratogenic effect in the pigeon is seen
at 9 mg/kg; in the chicken at 20 mg/kg; in the duck at
7 mg/kg. The chemical is a cholinesterase inhibitor
easily absorbed through the skin.

Disposal of Spills: The chemical should be absorbed
with paper towels placed in a plastic bag and burned
openly with the help of a flammable solvent. When placed
in a furnace, equal parts of sand or crushed limestone
should be added before covering with the solvent and
then igniting from a safe distance.

Manufacture: Technical grade Demeton is produced by
the reaction of diethyl phosphorochloridothionate with
2-ethyltriidoethanol in the presence of hydrochloric
acid. In the process, particularly at high temperature,
the thionate produced is isomerized to the thiolate and
the preparation contains a mixture of the two isomers.

Parathion

Parathion, marketed as Folidol, Thiophos and E605,
is correctly called dimethyl p-nitrophenyl phosphorothionate and is one of the most toxic, and was one of
the most widely used, organophosphorus insecticides.
Its methyl homolog is methylparathion where the ethyl
groups are substituted with methyls. The use of these
chemicals is now prohibited in some countries because
of their high toxicity. The chemical structure is as
follows:

$$(C_2H_5O)_2\ \overset{\displaystyle S}{\overset{\|}{P}}-O-\underset{}{\left\langle\!\!\!\bigcirc\!\!\!\right\rangle}-NO_2$$

Parathion is manufactured by the condensation of diethyl phosphorochlorothionate with sodium p-nitrophenate.

The purity of the product varies and an intermediate condensation product, ethyl phosphorothioate, may be present in up to 20% concentration.

Pure parathion is a pale yellow liquid with a molecular weight of 291.7, specific gravity of 1.26, boiling point of 375°C and a melting point of 6°C. It is highly soluble in most organic solvents except the alkanes but its solubility in water is only 24 ppm. It is relatively stable in neutral or acid but is rapidly hydrolyzed in alkaline solutions. In the environment, parathion is fairly persistent and may remain as the intact molecule on plants for a number of days. In addition, one of its major products of degradation is the formation of paroxon, which is an active form of parathion and is an even stronger cholinesterase inhibitor than the parent compound. Paroxon has an LD_{50} of 2.5 mg/kg.

The threshold limit value for skin has been set at 110 mcg/m^3. The LD_{50} in rats is 7 mg/kg. The LD50 of methylparathion is 25 mg/kg.

Phosmet

Phosmet, commonly marketed as Imidan or Prolate, chemically is dimethyl S-phthalimidomethyl phosphorothionate. The chemical structure is as follows:

$$(CH_3O)_2 \ PSCH_2N \underset{\overset{\|}{O}}{\overset{\overset{\|}{O}}{<}} \begin{matrix} C \\ \\ C \end{matrix}$$

Phosmet is manufactured by reaction of sodium dimethylphosphorodithioate and N-chloromethylphthalimide. The phosmet is an off-white crystal with a very offensive odor. It has a melting point of 72°C. It is soluble in most organic solvents except aliphatic hydrocarbons and the solubility in water is only 25 ppm. The half-life in aqueous solutions varies with the pH. At pH 4.5, 7.0, and 8.3, the half-life is 13 days, 12 hours, and four hours respectively. The persistence in soil, therefore,

varies with the make-up of the soil depending upon moisture and microbial population. The chemical is only
moderately toxic with an acute LD_{50} in male rats of
230 mg/kg. When ingested, phosmet is rapidly degraded
and excreted with metabolic studies in rats demonstrating
79% of the dose eliminated via the urine and 19% of the
dose eliminated via the feces. It is hydrolyzed to a
water soluble product as the predominant metabolic path-
way for degradation.

Azinphosmethyl and Azinphosethyl

Azinphosmethyl, commonly marketed as Guthion or
Gusathion, and azinphosethyl, commonly marketed as
Ethylguthion or Gusathion-A, are commonly used insecticides for fruit and vegetable crops. The chemical structure is as follows:

R = CH_3 azinphosmethyl
R = C_2H_5 azinphosethyl

The distinction between the azinphosmethyl and azinphosethyl is simply the substitution of a methyl or an
ethyl group. The compounds are synthesized by the condensation of corresponding dialkyl phosphorodithioate
with N-chloromethylbenzazimide. The azinphosmethyl is a
white crystalline substance with a melting point of
about $73^{\circ}C$. It is soluble in most organic solvents but
the water solubility is only 29 ppm. At elevated temperatures, it decomposes into a gas. Under natural conditions, however, the azinphos chemicals have a long residual activity. The azinphosethyl has a melting point of
$53^{\circ}C$.

Azinphosmethyl and azinphosethyl both have high mammalian toxicity. The acute oral LD_{50} for rats for the methyl
and ethyl homologs is 15 and 17.5 mg/kg respectively.
The TLV for skin has been set at 0.2 mg/m^3.

Diazinon

Diazinon, marketed as Basudin, Serolex, Neocydol, Nucidol and Spectracide, is chemically correctly a diethyl phosphorothionate. The chemical structure is as follows:

$$(C_2H_5O)_2 \; \overset{\overset{\displaystyle S}{\|}}{P} - O - \underset{\underset{\displaystyle N}{}}{\overset{\overset{\displaystyle CH_3}{|}}{\ }} N - CH(CH_3)_2$$

The chemical is produced beginning with the condensation of acetoacetate ester with isobutylamidine. In the pure form, diazinon is a colorless liquid, however, the usual physical state for use has a light amber to dark brown color. It has a boiling point of $89^{\circ}C$. It is highly soluble in most organic solvents but only soluble to 40 ppm in water. It is relatively unstable in acid in contrast to many organophosphates. The molecular weight is 204.38, the density is 1.11 at $23^{\circ}C$. Vapor pressure is 1.4×10^{-4} mm Hg at $20^{\circ}C$.

Diazinon is not only widely used in agriculture but is also widely used in structures for pest control. It is synergistic with the pyrethrins. The technical product of diazinon varies considerably by batch as the result of impurities. The oral LD_{50} for rats, therefore, is also reported at variable numbers from 108–250 mg/kg. The threshold limit value is set at 0.1 mg/m^3.

The chemical is rapidly metabolized in mammals and is excreted principally through the urine as a pyrimidinol or as desethyl diazinon.

The insecticide, diazinon, is a chemical which is commonly used within structures such as homes. Important to this type of use are levels of residues which might be found after normal application. The method of application has some significance since aerosol-type spray has a lower amount and duration of residue than insecticides applied by compressed air sprayer. Less movement of insecticide will occur to non-target areas with aerosol type spraying than with compressed air spraying, presumably because of less movement of the insecticide into the atmosphere by volatilization after application (Wright, 1975).

After applying diazinon as an aerosol into cracks
and crevices of rooms, no diazinon was found on floor
surfaces 48 hours after treatment (Wright, 1976). In
another study where technical diazinon was sprayed into
three apartments and into apartments which were fogged,
significantly more diazinon was found in those apartments
which were sprayed. There was no detectable diazinon
residue on plates taken from rooms four days after treatment by either sprayed or fogged application method
(Wright, 1974). Food areas, after being sprayed with
1-2% diazinon were found to have residues in the range
of 0.025-0.05 ppm. These levels were found one half hour
after treatment. All checks of residues at five hours
after treatment were below detectable levels of 0.01 ppm
(Jackson, 1975). Similarly, porcelain saucers which were
sprayed with diazinon and then analyzed for insecticide
residues for up to 28 days after spraying showed significant residues were greatly reduced within one day after
treatment. The calculations indicated that the maximum
amount of insecticide present on top of the dishes on the
day of exposure was less than 1/1,000 of the LD_{50} for
rats (Wright, 1971). Studies on levels of insecticide
which might be found in air after application have not
been performed.

Chloropyrifos

Chloropyrifos, commonly marketed as Dursban, Kill-
master or Lorsban, has the chemical name of diethyl
3,5,6-trichloro-2-pyridyl phosphorothionate. The structural formula is as follows:

$$(C_2H_5O)_2 \ \overset{\displaystyle S}{\underset{\displaystyle \|}{P}} - O - \text{(3,5,6-trichloro-2-pyridyl)}$$

The chemical is a white granular crystal with a melting point of 42°C. It is highly soluble in most organic
solvents but not in water. The density is 1.398 at 43°C,
molecular weight is 350.59, the vapor pressure is
1.87×10^{-5} mm Hg at 25°C. It has a mild mercaptan odor.
It is quite stable at room temperature with decomposition

occurring above 163°C and hydrolysis occurring under strong alkaline conditions. The chemical has an acute LD_{50} for rats at 163 mg/kg. It is rapidly metabolized and excreted mainly in the urine with the degradation product appearing mainly due to dealkylation. About 80% of the metabolites in the urine consist of trichloro-pyridyl phosphate.

It is widely used in agriculture and in structure pest control. In the latter, it is principally a contact toxicant with typical spray formulations varying in concentration from 0.25-0.5% spray.

Trichlorfon

Trichlorfon, commonly marketed as Dipterex, Dylox, Anthon or Neguvon, chemically is 0,0-dimethyl (2,2,2-trichloro-1-hydroxyethyl) phosphate. The structural formula is as follows:

$$CH_3O \diagdown \atop CH_3O \diagup P - CH - \underset{\underset{Cl}{|}}{\overset{\overset{OH}{|}}{C}} - Cl$$

The chemical is used for a variety of insecticidal purposes in both agriculture and in structures. It is commonly a white crystal. It has a molecular weight of 257.5, specific gravity of 1.73 at 20°C, melting point of 83°C and boiling point of 100°C. It is soluble in water, benzene, chloroform and ether but is insoluble in oils. The vapor pressure is 7.8×10^{-6} mm Hg at 20°C. At high temperature and low pH, the chemical is decomposed to form dichlorvos (DDVP).

The chemical has an LD_{50} of 400-500 mg/kg in rats. It is more toxic to birds with an LD_{50} of 40 mg/kg. It is also toxic to fish. No TLV's have been established. In July of 1979, it came under RPAR review.

The chemical is known to exist in the environment for long periods of time in water. It has been noted to be present for as long as 526 days after application and at room temperatures of 20°C. It is, therefore, not to be used in conditions where run-off may occur.

Naled

Naled, marketed commercially as Dibrom, is correctly called 1,2-dibromo-2,2-dichloroethyl dimethyl phosphate. The structural formula is as follows:

$$(CH_3O)_2 \underset{\overset{\|}{O}}{P} - OCHBrCBrCl_2$$

Naled is manufactured by the bromination of dichlorvos. The pure material melts at $26^\circ C$. The chemical has a boiling point of $110^\circ C$. It is insoluble in water but readily soluble in most organic solvents except aliphatic hydrocarbons. The chemical is somewhat more stable than dichlorvos, however, it is completely hydrolyzed in water within two days at room temperature. The toxicity to mammals is considered relatively low with the oral LD_{50} to rats at 430 mg/kg. The chemical is used as a short lived insecticide on vegetable crops and for fly and mosquito control. Breakdown is prevented in some commercial formulations by the addition of phosphoric acid as a stabilizer. The chemical is readily degraded in most mammals. By reacting with natural thio compounds, naled also transforms readily into dichlorvos, which may be the actual insecticide in the environment.

Malathion

Malathion is commonly marketed under the tradenames Cythion, Karbofos, Malaphos, Malathiozol, Malphos and others. Structurally, it belongs to the organophosphates of the phosphorodithioate type and chemically is a dimethyl phosphorothiolothionate. The structural formula is as follows:

$$(CH_3O)_2 \underset{\overset{\|}{S}}{P} - S - CH - \underset{\overset{\|}{O}}{C}OC_2H_5$$
$$\overset{|}{C}H_2\underset{\overset{\|}{O}}{C}OC_2H_5$$

It is manufactured by the addition of dimethyl hydrogen phosphorodithioate to diethyl maleate. The chemical is a yellow liquid with a boiling point of 120°C and a specific gravity of 1.23. Solubility in water is 145 ppm at 20°C. It is highly soluble in most organic solvents. It is rapidly hydrolyzed in aqueous solutions above a pH of 7 or below a pH of 5. This means that it has a very narrow range of stability in the environment. It will also decompose if stored in contact with activated iron, tin plate, lead or copper. The chemical is only slightly soluble in water at 145 ppm although it is miscible in many organic solvents. Highly refined petroleum oils, which are frequently used as insecticide solvents, will dissolve less than 1% malathion. It is soluble in alcohols, ethers, ketones, esters and fatty oils. The chemical has a low toxicity with an oral LD_{50} for rats ranging from 600-1400 mg/kg. The dermal LD_{50} for rats is greater than 4400 mg/kg. The TLV for skin is 10 mg/m^3.

Although a compound of low toxicity, several disadvantages have become apparent. As mentioned, the chemical has a very low range of stability in regard to aqueous pH. It is also highly toxic to fish, bees and a variety of non-target arthropods. Finally, following general and continued use, resistance can almost always be anticipated. Impurities also exist in the manufacture which apparently increase during shipment or storage in warm areas. On the other hand, malathion residues are lost fairly rapidly after application and the chemical is considered to be ineffective 10-14 days following use.

Toxicity of malathion is direct although considered low in most susceptible insects. However, bioactivation in the form of the production of the oxon can occur in insects. Detoxification occurs principally via the route of demethylation. Detoxification also occurs by breakdown of the carboxy ester groups on the chemical via the carboxyesterase enzyme. This is a major route of detoxification in mammals.

Tetrachlorvinphos

Tetrachlorvinphos is marketed as Gardona or Rabon. This chemical is synthesized by the Perkow reaction from methylphosphite and 2,4,5,α,α-pentachloroacetophenone. The structural formula is as follows:

$$(CH_3O)_2 \underset{\underset{ClCH}{\|}}{\overset{\overset{O}{\|}}{P}} - O - \overset{\|}{C} - \text{(ring: Cl, Cl, Cl)}$$

The melting point of the two isomers formed are 62°C
and 98°C. Technical Gardona is a white crystalline solid
with a melting point of about 97°C. It contains 98% of
the B-isomers. Solubility in water is very limited,
11 ppm at 20°C. It is soluble in most organic solvents
except hydrocarbons. It is considered to be very low in
toxicity with an oral LD_{50} for rats at 4,000 mg/kg and
rats have been fed a maximum of 125 ppm for two years
without harmful effects.

Methidathion

Methidathion, marketed as Supracide or Ustracide, is
a chemical with the general formula of a dimethyl phosphorothiolothionate. The structural formula is as
follows:

$$(CH_3O)_2 \overset{\overset{S}{\|}}{P} S - CH_2 - N \underset{N = C - OCH_3}{\overset{C - S}{\diagup}}$$

The chemical is a colorless crystalline substance with
a melting point of 39-40°C. It is readily soluble in
acetone, benzene and ethanol and the solubility in water
is 240 ppm at 25°C. It is stable in neutral or acid
media but is readily hydrolyzed in alkali.

Mammalian toxicity in rats is 25-50 mg/kg. The chemical is degraded in the environment by hydrolysis.

Methamidophos

Methamidophos, commonly marketed as Monitor or Camaron, is correctly called O,S,dimethyl phosphoramidothiolate. The structural formula is as follows:

$$CH_3O \diagdown \quad O$$
$$\underset{H_2N \diagup}{P} - SCH_3$$

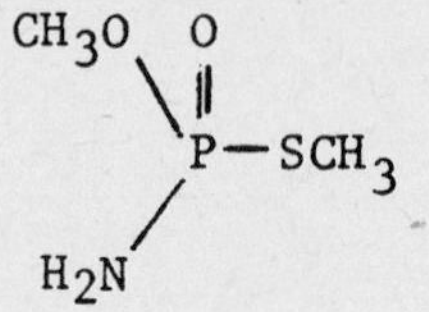

This is a highly active insecticidal compound with a broad spectrum of use, particularly effective in controlling caterpillers in the field. The chemical is a colorless crystalline solid with a melting point of 44.5°C. It is readily soluble in water, alcohols, ketones and aliphatic hydrocarbons and only slightly soluble or insoluble in ethers. The chemical has a very high mammalian toxicity with an acute oral LD$_{50}$ for rats of about 30 mg/kg. In spite of the high toxicity, it has only a weak in vitro anticholinesterase activity.

The N-acetyl derivative of methamidophos is named acephate and has frequently replaced this insecticide because of its lower toxicity.

Acephate

Acephate, commonly marketed as Orthene or Ortran, is correctly called O,S-dimethyl N-acetylphosphoramidothiolate. The structural formula is as follows:

$$CH_3O \diagdown \quad O \qquad\qquad O$$
$$\underset{CH_3S \diagup}{P} - NH - CCH_3$$

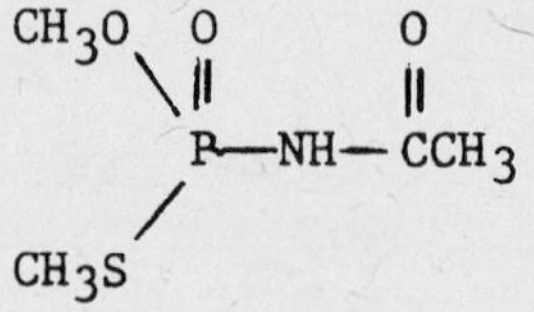

Acephate is the N-acetyl derivative of the insecticide methamidophos. It is a white crystalline powder with a melting point of 91°C and is highly soluble in water to about 65%. The acetylation of the parent compound causes a striking decrease in mammalian toxicity with the oral LD$_{50}$ for mice and rats being 360 and 945 mg/kg respec-

tively. This compares with the LD_{50} for mice of methamidophos of 27 mg/kg.

Phorate

Phorate, commonly marketed as Thimet, is a diethyl
phosphorothiolothionate. The chemical structure is as
follows:

$$\underset{(C_2H_5O)_2}{} \overset{\displaystyle S}{\underset{\displaystyle \|}{P}}SCH_2SC_2H_5$$

Phorate is a liquid with a boiling point of 100°C.
The specific gravity is 1.535. Phorate has a high mammalian toxicity and the LD_{50} for rats is only 2-4 mg/kg.
It is a systemic insecticide. The chemical is unstable
to hydrolysis and the half-life at pH 8 at 70°C, a high
temperature, is two hours. It protects plants for a
long time because the degradation product, in the form
of a sulfoxide metabolite, can persist in plants and in
soils.

Oxydemeton-Methyl

Oxydemeton-methyl is commonly marketed as Metasystox R.
The chemical structure is as follows:

$$(CH_3O)_2 \;\; \overset{\displaystyle O}{\underset{\displaystyle \|}{P}}SCH_2CH_2\overset{\displaystyle O}{\underset{\displaystyle \uparrow}{S}}C_2H_5$$

The chemical is a systemic insecticide. It is a
clear amber liquid with a boiling point of 106°C. The
specific gravity is 1.28. The chemical is miscible with
water and soluble in most organic solvents except petroleum ether. It is relatively stable under alkaline conditions and is, therefore, compatible with alkaline
pesticides. It has an oral LD_{50} for rats of 70 mg/kg.

The methyl homolog is marketed as Metasystox S. This
chemical is similar except that the oral LD_{50} for rats is
105 mg/kg.

Azodrin

Azodrin is an organophosphate with a molecular formula of $C_7H_{14}NO_5P$. The structural formula is as follows:

$$(CH_3O)_2PO.OC(CH_3)=CH.CO.NH.CH_3$$

Azodrin is the dimethyl phosphate ester of 3-hydroxy-N-methyl-cis-crotonamide. It is marketed under the names Monocrotophos, Monocron and Nuvacron. In the Pacific Northwest it finds its major use on potatoes. It is marketed as an insecticide and acaracide on cotton, potatoes, peanuts and ornamentals and is used as an insecticide on tobacco and sugar cane.

The manufacturing process is the reaction of trimethyl-phosphite with methyl N-methyl-methyl-2-chloroacetamide.

The chemical is very soluble in water, alcohol and acetone and only slightly soluble in petrochemicals such as kerosene or diesel fuel. It is a crystalline or reddish-brown semi-solid. It hydrolyzes rapidly above a pH of 7 and when stored has a half-life of 22 days at a pH of 7 or less. It is quite corrosive, particularly to iron although not to glass, aluminum or stainless steel. The solid has a melting point of 54°C and a boiling point of 125°C.

The chemical is considered quite toxic with an oral LD_{50} in rats of 21 mg/kg and in mice of 15 mg/kg. It is toxic to trout and bluegill at 12 ppm/24 hours and 23 ppm/24 hours respectively. Birds are quite susceptible with toxicity listed at 3-4 mg/kg. The chemical is listed as dangerously flammable and careful storage is recommended. It is relatively stable in the environment with 50% being found present after a period of 21 days. Nevertheless, the re-entry time is currently listed at 48 hours.

In animals, the chemical can be analyzed directly by chromatography methods. The analysis of urine of experimental animals indicates that the chemical is metabolized by hydrolysis to N-hydroxymethylamide.

Animal toxicity experiments have demonstrated no effect in the diet with two year feedings to rats at a 1 ppm level and a 1.6 ppm level to dogs. Feeding studies also performed for 90 days at levels of 135 ppm produced no histopathological effects.

Ethion

Ethion is an organophosphate used principally as an acaricide. The molecular formula is $C_{19}H_{22}O_4P_2S_4$ and the structural formula is as follows:

$$
\begin{array}{cc}
\quad\quad\quad S & \quad\quad S \\
C_2H_5O \quad \| & \| \quad OC_2H_5 \\
\qquad\qquad\searrow P.S.CH_2.S.P\searrow \\
C_2H_5O^{\nearrow} & \quad\quad OC_2H_5
\end{array}
$$

The chemical is also known as Diethion, Nialate, Phosphotox E and Rodocide.

In the Pacific Northwest, it is used principally as an acaricide for the control of aphids, thrips, scale and so forth.

The chemical has a molecular weight of 384.48 and a density of 1.20 at $20^{\circ}C$. The melting point is -12 to $-13^{\circ}C$ and it has a very low vapor pressure of 1.5×10^{-6} mm Hg at $25^{\circ}C$. In the pure form it is a colorless liquid. The chemical is non-corrosive and has a long shelf life although it is slowly oxidized in air. It is only slightly soluble in water but is soluble in a variety of organic solvents such as xylene, chloroform, kerosene and other petroleum oils. In rats, the oral LD_{50} is 13 mg/kg and the percutaneous LD_{50} is 62 mg/kg. It is very toxic to aquatic life. Long-term feeding experiments in female rats fed 300 ppm in their diet for 28 days caused no deaths although cholinesterase inhibition occurred at levels above 10 ppm.

In checking environmental samples for residues, laboratory methods preferred are thin layer chromatography or gas chromatography.

References

Abou-Donia, M.B. (1979) Delayed neurotoxicity of phenyl-phosphonothioate esters. Science 205:713-715.

Bouldin, T.W. and J.B. Cavanagh (1979) Organophosphorous neuropathy. Amer J Pathol 94:241-270.

Brown, H.W. (1971) Electroencephalographic changes and disturbance of brain function following human organophosphate exposure. NW Med 39:845-846.

Burkart, J.A., D.Y. Takade and R. Potter (1977)
Estimates of variability in a comparative standardized
cholinesterase assay. Bull Environ Contam Toxicol
18:89-95.

Davignon, L.F., J. St-Pierre, G. Charest and F.J.
Tourangeau (1965) A study of the chronic effects
of insecticides in man. Can Med Assoc J 92:597-602.

Derache, F. (1977) Organophosphorus pesticides; criteria
(dose/effect relationships) for organophosphorus
pesticides. Report of a Working Group of Experts
prepared for the Commission of the European Communities, Directorate-General for Social Affairs,
Health and Safety Directorate. Pergamon Press,
Oxford.

Dille, J.R. and P.W. Smith (1964) Central nervous
system effects of chronic exposure to organophosphate
insecticides. Aerospace Med 34:475-478.

Duffy, F.H., J.L. Burchfiel, P.H. Bartels, M. Gaon and
V.M. Sim (1979) Long-term effects of an organophos-
phate upon the human electroencephalogram. Toxicol
Appl Pharmacol 47:161-176.

Durham, W.F., H.R. Wolfe and G.E. Quinby (1965)
Organophosphorus insecticides and mental alertness.
Arch Environ Health 10:55-66.

Environmental Protection Agency (1974) Farm workers
dealing with pesticides. Fed Regis 39:9457-9462.

Fenichel, G.M., W.B. Kibler, W.H. Olson and W.D. Dettbarn
(1972) Chronic inhibition of cholinesterase as a
cause of myopathy. Neurol 22:1026-1033.

Gadoth, N. and A. Fisher (1978) Late onset of neuromuscular block in organophosphorus poisoning.
Ann Intern Med 88:654-655.

Harrell, M., J.J. Shea and J.R. Emmett (1978) Bilateral
sudden deafness following combined insecticide
poisoning. Laryngoscope 88:1348-1351.

Hayes, M.M.M., N.G. Van Der Westhuizen and M. Gelfan
(1978) Organophosphate poisoning in Rhodesia.
South African Med J 54:230-234.

Hierons, R. and M.K. Johnson (1978) Clinical and
toxicological investigations of a case of delayed
neuropathy in man after acute poisoning by an
organophosphorus pesticide. Arch Toxicol 40:279-284.

Howard, J.K., N.J. East and J.L. Chaney (1978)
Plasma cholinesterase activity in early pregnancy.
Arch Environ Health 33:277.

Ikuta, S. (1973) A case of acute intoxication by an
organophosphorus pesticide. J Jap Ass Rural Med
22:113.

Ishikawa, S. (1973) Chronic optic neuropathy due to
environmental exposure to organophosphorus pesticides.
J Jap Ophthalmol Soc 77:1835-1886.

Ishikawa, S. (1978) Ocular manifestations by chronic
organophosphate pesticide intoxication. Excerpta
Med Int Congr Ser 442:31.

Jackson, M.D. and C.G. Wright (1975) Diazinon and
chlorpyrifos residues in food after insecticidal
treatment in room. Bull Environ Contam Toxicol
13:593-595.

Johnson, M.K. (1975a) The delayed neuropathy caused by
some organophosphorus esters: Mechanism and challenge.
CRC Crit Rev Toxicol 3:289-316.

Johnson, M.K. (1975b) Organophosphorus esters causing
delayed neurotoxic effects. Arch Toxicol 34:250-288.

Jusic, A. and S. Milic (1978) Neuromuscular synapse
testing in two cases of suicidal organophosphorous
pesticide poisoning. Arch Environ Health 33:240.

Knaak, J.B., K.T. Maddy, T. Jackson, A.S. Fredrickson,
S.A. Peoples and R. Love (1978) Cholinesterase
activity in blood samples collected from field
workers and non-field workers in California.
Toxicol Appl Pharmacol 45:755-770.

Knaak, J.B., K.T. Maddy and S. Khalifa (1979) Alkyl
   phosphate metabolite levels in the urine of field
   workers giving blood for cholinesterase test in
   California. Bull Environ Contam Toxicol 21:375-380.

Kraus, J.F., D.M. Richards, N.O. Borhani, R. Mull,
   W.W. Kilgore and W. Winterlin (1977) Physiological
   response to organophosphate residues in field workers.
   Arch Environ Contam Toxicol 5:471-485.

Lores, E.M., D.E. Bradway and R.F. Moseman (1978)
   Organophosphorus pesticide poisonings in humans:
   Determination of residues and metabolites in tissues
   and urine. Arch Environ Health 33:270-276.

Lotti, M. and M.K. Johnson (1978) Neurotoxicity of
   organophosphorus pesticides: Predictions can be based
   on in vitro studies with hen and human enzymes.
   Arch Toxicol 41:215-221.

Maibach, H.I., R.J. Feldmann, T.H. Milby and W.F. Serat
   (1971) Regional variations in percutaneous penetration in man. Arch Environ Health 23:208-211.

Michel, H.O. (1949) An electrometric method for the
   determination of red blood cell and plasma cholinesterase activity. J Lab Clin Med 34:1564-1568.

Milby, T.H. (ed.) (1974) Occupational exposure to
   pesticides. Report to the Federal Working Group on
   Pest Management from the Task Group on Occupational
   Exposure to Pesticides. Washington, DC.

Morgan, J.P. and P. Penovich (1978) Jamaica ginger
   paralysis. Arch Neurol 35:530-532.

Nabb, D.P. and F. Whitfield (1967) Determination of
   cholinesterase by automated pH-stat method. Arch
   Environ Health 15:147-154.

Namba, T., C.T. Nolte, J. Jackrel and D. Groh (1971)
   Poisoning due to organophosphate insecticides.
   Amer J Med 50:475-491.

National Technical Information Service (1976) Pesticide
   induced delayed neuropathy. Proceedings of a Conference held in Washington, DC, February 19-20.

Owens, C.B., E.W. Owens and D. Zahn (1978) The extent of exposure of migrant workers to pesticide and pesticide residues. Int J Chronobiol 5:428-429.

Rayner, M.D., J.S. Popper, E.W. Carvalho and R. Hurov (1972) Hyporeflexia in workers chronically exposed to organophosphate insecticides. Res Commun Chem Pathol Pharmacol 4:596-606.

Rodnitzky, R.L., H.A. Levin and D.L. Mick (1975) Occupational exposure to organophosphate pesticides. Arch Environ Health 30:98.

Rowntree, D.W., S. Nevin and A. Wilson (1950) The effects of diisopropylfluorophosphonate in schizophrenia and manic depressive psychosis. J Neurol Neurosurg Psychiat 13:47-59.

Sidell, F.R. (1974) Soman and sarin: Clinical manifestations and treatment of accidental poisoning by organophosphates. Clin Toxicol 7:1-17.

Stalberg, E, P. Hilton-Brown, B. Kolmodin-Hedman, B. Holmstedt and K.B. Augustinsson (1978) Effect of occupational exposure to organophosphorus insecticides on neuromuscular function. Scand J Work Environ Health 4:255-261.

Tabershaw, I.R. and W.C. Cooper (1966) Sequelae of acute organic phosphate poisoning. J Occup Med 8:5-20.

Tamura, O. (1978) Organophosphorus pesticides as a cause of myopia in school children: An epidemiological study. Excerpta Med Int Congr Ser 442:31.

Uchida, T. (1974) A case of retinochoroid pathosis due to chronic intoxication by organophosphorus pesticides. Jap Rev Clin Ophthalmol 68:191-192.

Vandekar, M. (1957) Anaesthetic effect produced by organophosphorus compounds. Nature 179:154-155.

Wadia, R.S., C. Sadagopan, R.B. Amin and H.V. Sardesai (1974) Neurological manifestations of organophosphorous insecticide poisoning. J Neurol Neurosurg Psychiat 37:841-847.

Willis, P.H. (1972) The measurement and significance of changes in cholinesterase activities of erythrocytes and plasma in man and animals. CRC Crit Rev Toxicol 5:153-202.

Wolfe, H.R., D.C. Staiff, J.F. Armstrong and J.E. Davis (1978) Exposure of fertilizer mixing plant workers to disulfoton. Bull Environ Contam Toxicol 20:79-86.

Wood, W., J. Gavica, H.W. Brown, M. Watson and W.W. Benson (1971) Implication of organophosphate pesticide poisoning in the plane crash of a duster pilot. Aerospace Med 41:1111-1113.

WHO (1978) Chemistry and specifications of pesticides. Second Report of the WHO Expert Committee on Vector Biology and Controls, World Health Organization, Technical Report Series #620, Geneva.

Wright, C.G. and M.D. Jackson (1971) Propoxur, chlordane and diazinon on porcelain china saucers after kitchen cabinet spraying. J Econ Entom 64:457-459.

Wright, C.G. and M.D. Jackson (1974) A comparison of residues produced by spraying and fogging of diazinon in buildings. Bull Environ Contam Toxicol 12:177-181.

Wright, C.G. and M.D. Jackson (1975) Insecticide residues in nontarget areas of rooms after two methods of crack and crevice application. Bull Environ Contam Toxicol 13:123-128.

Wright, C.G. and M.D. Jackson (1976) Insecticide movement following application to crevices in rooms. Arch Environ Contam Toxicol 14:492-500.

Yager, J., H. McLean, M. Hudes and R.C. Spear (1976) Components of variability in blood cholinesterase assay results. J Occup Med 18:242-244.

5

Carbamates and
Ethylenebisdithiocarbamates

Introduction

The carbamate compounds are a class of cholinesterase inhibiting pesticides or fungicides with the general chemical structure of

$$\begin{array}{c} H \\ \diagdown \\ H_3C \diagup \end{array} N - \overset{\displaystyle O}{\overset{\displaystyle \|}{C}} - O - R$$

Examples of commonly used commercial products are aldicarb (Temik), methomyl (Lannate), propoxur (Baygon) and carbaryl (Sevin).

The following section is divided into two parts. Aldicarb is discussed as an example of a typical carbamate pesticide along with others. Utilized principally as a fumigant, the ethylenebisdithiocarbamates, however, have been under RPAR because a breakdown product, ethylenethiourea (ETU) is a suspect teratogen and carcinogen. The ethylenebisdithiocarbamates are dealt with in a separate section of this chapter.

247

Aldicarb

Production and Use

Aldicarb is a carbamate pesticide with a broad spectrum of effectiveness against a variety of insects, mites or nematodes. The chemical is manufactured under the trade-name of Temik. It is used principally in the South and in the Pacific Northwest on crops such as cotton, sugar beets, potatoes, peanuts, and on ornamentals. The chemical formula is

$$
\begin{array}{ccc}
CH_3 & & O \\
| & & \| \\
CH_3-S-C \!\!-\!\!-\!\!- C\!\!=\!\!N\!\!-\!\!O\!\!-\!\!C\!\!-\!\!N\!\!-\!\!CH_3 \\
| & | & | \\
CH_3 & H & H
\end{array}
$$

Impurities present in the manufactured product include dimethylurea, a propionitrile and a propionaldehyde.

The Physical and Chemical Properties

The molecular weight is 190.2. At room temperature it is a white, odorless crystal with a melting point of 100°C. The vapor pressure is 1×10^{-4} mm Hg at 25°C. The chemical is soluble in a variety of organic solvents, principally acetone, chloroform, ethanol and methylene chloride. It is virtually insoluble in water.

Animal Toxicology Studies

A short, ten day feeding study in chickens demonstrated death with dosages at 2.5 mg/kg/day but no ill effects at 1 mg/kg/day. The number of animals used was small and only general conclusions concerning a rough figure for development of a fairly acute intoxication can be developed from this study (Schlinke, 1977). Similarly, Schlinke fed calves and sheep aldicarb in a dosage of 0.10 mg/kg. This led to toxic symptoms and depression of cholinesterase. In addition, although a dosage of 0.05 mg/kg did not lead to clinical symptoms, there was an 85% depression of cholinesterase in 96 hours. In

sheep, dosages of 1.0 mg/kg led to clinical symptoms of
intoxication with a 91% drop in cholinesterase by six
hours. With a dose of 0.25 mg/kg, no clinical symptoms
were noted, however, a 52% drop in cholinesterase occurred within six hours.

Metabolism

Aldicarb, a carbamate ester of an oxime, is an unusual
insecticide in that it does not contain an aromatic
moiety. In general, the metabolism of aldicarb in plants,
insects and mammals is the same. The metabolic reaction
of aldicarb in cotton plants is to oxidize the chemical
to the sulfoxide and then more slowly to the sulfone.
The former is relatively stable in plants and is a major
intact metabolite present after treatment. The sulfoxide
has a higher anticholinesterase activity than aldicarb
proper and it is possible that systemic intoxication may
be secondary to this breakdown product. Eventually, a
number of sulfoxide metabolic products develop in plants.
Rats given oral sub-lethal dosages of aldicarb rapidly
metabolize the chemical and excrete it principally in the
urine. Small amounts of nitrile sulfoxide and nitrile
sulfone are also formed. In general, the metabolism of
aldicarb in plants and in the rat are similar but the
rates of degradation vary.
Aldicarb fed to a lactating cow is rapidly eliminated
in the urine, e.g. 83% of a single oral dose after 24
hours. Some metabolites are also found in the milk (3%
of applied dose). The milk of cows given aldicarb on a
daily basis for 14 days at a dose equivalent to 0.12,
0.6 and 1.2 ppm in the feed contained, on a daily average, 4.4 and 7.3 ppb, 25.6 and 35.9 ppb, and 43.6 and
66.5 ppb of the major metabolites. The overall spectrum
of metabolites on a long-term feeding basis is the same
as the case of single oral treatment.
The metabolism of the carbamate insecticides in general, including aldicarb, has been summarized by Fukuto
(1972).

Environmental Fate

Aldicarb is fairly persistent in soil following application to fields. Residues can be detected in the soil
as well as in crops which are grown on treated fields.

On treated areas, residues up to 42 ppm have been detected
after seven days, then dropping off to 2.75 ppm after 43
days. Animals from fields under investigation have also
been studied. In a study of 14 birds, one whole body
residue consisted of 0.07 ppm. Studies on the livers of
eight mammals trapped in the field area under study did
not reveal any residue of aldicarb and/or its metabolites
(Woodham, 1973).

Teratogenicity

Aldicarb has been fed to rats in dosages which are
almost equal to the LD_{50} without any evidence of teratogenicity.

Carcinogenicity

Animals have been tested for carcinogenicity by treating hair-free skin of mice. The results of this test
were negative.

Mutagenicity

Aldicarb is a suspected mutagen. Studies by Blevins,
Lijinsky and Regan (1977) suggest that the chemical can
become mutagenic when converted to a nitroso derivative.
Under these circumstances, breaks are apparent in DNA.
Aldicarb alone does not produce there effects. The
suggestion is that if aldicarb were nitrosated after
ingestion or by some other natural product, the chemical
might then become a mutagen.
    Seiler (1977) in studies on bone marrow nuclei was
unable to demonstrate changes with pesticide alone.
Again, if nitroso ethylenethiourea was given along with
the pesticide, micronucleic changes were seen in a dose-
response type of relationship following intraperitoneal
injection and with an apparent no-efect level at 15-18
mg/kg. In the same series of experiments, aldicarb was
positive in the Ames test. Seiler concludes from his
experiments with agricultural chemicals plus sodium
nitrate that mutagenic events stemming from N-nitrosation
could be regarded as small providing that the micro
nucleus test system was a good indicator for mutagenicity
(which was questioned). Nitrosation did not proceed in

man any more than in the mouse and germ cells are not
more susceptible to the nitroso compounds than somatic
cells. In short, the question of mutagenicity of the
chemical is not clearly settled.

Human Toxicology

   The clinical experience with aldicarb intoxication is
extremely limited. Two outbreaks of illness occurred in
Nebraska (MMWR, 1979) which were associated with the consumption of hydroponic cucumbers (grown in water). The
symptoms were typical of carbamate and/or organophosphate
intoxication and in the two episodes, a total of 14 individuals became sick with symptoms occurring within 15-135
minutes after ingestion of the cucumbers. The ill persons, eight females and six males, ranged in age from six
to 80 years. The length of illness was approximately
five to six hours and none of the patients received
specific medical treatment although all recovered quickly
and completely. The symptoms are listed below.

	Illness I	Illness II
Diarrhea	100%	100%
Nausea/vomiting	89	100
Perspiration	89	100
Blurred vision	75	60
Abdominal pain	67	100
Muscle fasciculation	56	80
Temporary paralysis	67	–
Headache	11	60

   Analysis of cucumbers grown at the particular laboratory (although the original cucumbers were obviously
consumed) showed that aldicarb was present in 6.7 and
10.7 ppm. The water-nutrient solution of the hydroponic
cucumbers was then analyzed and found to contain 1.8 ppm
aldicarb. The source of the aldicarb contamination was
never determined. The case may represent an example of
aldicarb, an insecticide intended for soil application,
developing a markedly toxic solution when mixed with
water.
   In a proprietary study, three groups of four adult
males were each given a dose of aldicarb corresponding
to 0.1, 0.05, or 0.025 mg/kg. Blood cholinesterase
levels were monitored before and after the dose as were

clinical symptoms. All four men, at the highest dose, developed mild cholinergic symptoms and at one hour, there was some slight depression of the serum cholinesterase. At six hours after the above dose, the cholinesterase levels of all groups were statistically similar.

Urine of employees working in production has been analyzed for evidence of the breakdown product, aldicarb sulfoxide. This may represent one means of demonstrating whether exposure has occurred - in addition to the serum cholinesterase monitoring.

For specific therapy of intoxication see the section on medical treatment of carbamates at the end of this chapter.

Methomyl

Methomyl, generically referred to as acetimidic acid, is a carbamate insecticide which is marketed under the tradenames of Lannate or Nudrin.

The molecular formula is $C_5H_{10}N_2O_2S$ and the structural formula is

$$CH_3.S.\overset{\overset{\displaystyle CH_3}{|}}{C} N.O.\overset{\overset{\displaystyle O}{\|}}{C}.NHCH_3$$

The chemical is manufactured by reacting an oxime with methyl isocyanate. Its major use in the Pacific Northwest is on sweet corn. It is also used extensively as an insecticide on vegetables and on tobacco, cotton, alfalfa and soybeans.

The chemical has a molecular weight of 162.2. It has a low volatility with a vapor pressure of $5x10^{-5}$ mm Hg at $25^{\circ}C$. It is manufactured as a crystal or as a white crystalline solid. It is stable in both the solid form and aqueous solutions and is particularly stable in neutral or slightly acetic solutions. It is soluble in water and most organic solvents and is commonly formulated with methanol, ethanol, isopropanol or acetone. Its melting point is 78-79$^{\circ}C$ and the density is 1.2946 at $24^{\circ}C$. It is non-corrosive in solution although it has a slightly sulfurous odor.

In experimental animals, the acute oral LD_{50} in rats is 17 mg/kg, the inhalation LC_{50} is 77 ppm and the LD_{50}

via percutaneous route is more than 1 g/kg. In monkeys, the lower limit of observable effect is 40 mg/kg and in birds is about 15 mg/kg.

Although there have been some reported incidents of possible occupational exposure problems, the chemical actually is readily metabolized and degraded in both mammals and the environment. It is likely that the cited cases may have had exposure to other organophosphates at the same time with either a synergistic effect or intoxication from other chemicals. The half-life in water is estimated to be five to six days. It is degraded rapidly in soil, principally to carbon dioxide. In mammals, the chemical seems to be degraded into carbon dioxide and acetonitrile. In addition, it may be that the degradation product seen in the urine may consist of oxime-O-sulfate, free oxime or oxime glucuronide.

Toxicology studies on experimental animals indicate that it does not have a cumulative action. The chemical does act as an anticholinesterase inhibitor, and although reversible, side effects of overdosage would be expected to be the same as an acute organophosphate intoxication. Three generation reproduction studies have been performed on rats fed 50-100 ppm and no adverse effects were noted. Teratogenic effects were not seen in rabbits fed up to 100 ppm during pregnancy. Mutagenic studies in bacteria have been negative although the concern remains for the nitroso derivatives as being a potential mutagen.

In humans, the chemical may cause acute cholinesterase inhibition which should be treated in the manner of other carbamates. The chemical is a skin irritant and may cause conjunctivitis or possibly other irritations of a mild nature of the mucous membranes. Residues perhaps may be detected by high pressure liquid chromatography. For specific therapy of intoxication see the section on medical treatment of carbamates at the end of this chapter.

Butylate

Butylate is a carbamate with the generic name S-ethyl diisobutylthiocarbamate. It is generally known under the tradename of Sutan. It is an herbicide with a molecular formula of $C_{11}H_{23}NOS$ and a structural formula of

$$C_2H_5S-\overset{\overset{\textstyle O}{\|}}{C}-N(CH_2-CH-(CH_3)_2)_2$$

It has a molecular weight of 217.4 and a specific gravity of 0.9402. Its boiling point is 71°C and it has relatively low volatility with a vapor pressure of 13×10^{-3} mm Hg at 25°C. The chemical is a liquid with an amber color. It is not very soluble in a variety of solvents. It is soluble in water only to 36 ppm. It is miscible in kerosene, xylene, acetone and ethyl alcohol.

The chemical is used as a selective herbicide to provide pre-emergence control of weeds. In the Pacific Northwest, it is used particularly on sweet corn crops. For best use under normal conditions, butylate must be mechanically incorporated into the soil to a depth of two to three inches. In the soil, microbial breakdown is the major mechanism of disappearance and the half-life of butylate under normal growing conditions is 1½–3 weeks. It is degraded to sulfoxide in the soil. In plants, the chemical disappears within 7–14 days, being rapidly metabolized to carbon dioxide, diisobutylamine, fatty acids and amines.

The acute LD_{50} in rats is 4,000 mg/kg and in rabbits is greater than 4,640 mg/kg. The 50% lethal concentration for fish varies from 4.2 to 7.2 ppm after 96 hours of exposure. Toxicity via the skin or inhalation is considered low. Long-term feeding experiments of 90 days in rats demonstrated no effect at 32 mg/kg/day and in dogs, no effect at 40 mg/kg/day. Metabolism in mammals would indicate that the chemical is degraded to a mercapturic acid. In rats, about 40% of an administered dose has been metabolized directly with formation of carbon dioxide.

Laboratory methods of analysis would include steam distillation followed by formation of a cupric dithiocarbamate complex. The chemical may also be analyzed by gas chromatography.

For specific therapy of intoxication see the section on medical treatment of carbamates at the end of this chapter.

Carbofuran

Carbofuran is a methylcarbamate acid with the generic name 2,2-dimethyl-2,3-dihydro-7-benzofuranyl. It is marketed under the tradename of Furadan. In the Pacific Northwest, it is used mainly in grain crops such as alfalfa. It is also used on other grain crops, particularly corn or tobacco. It is generally applied at a dosage of 0.25–1.0 kg/hectare (0.5–2.0 lb/acre).

The chemical has a molecular formula of $C_{12}H_{15}NO_3$ and a structural formula of

The melting point is 150-152°C and the density is 1.180 at 20°C. Vapor pressure is 2×10^{-5} mm Hg at 33°C. The chemical is soluble in water at 700 ppm at 25°C. It is also soluble in a variety of organic solvents such as acetone, benzene, dimethylformanide and DMSO. The technical product is a white crystalline solid which is odorless. It is stable under neutral or acid conditions but unstable in alkaline media. It has a stable shelf life and is noncorrosive and nonflammable.

In the environment, the chemical has a half-life estimated in various soils as being from 30-60 days. On plants, no traces of the chemical have been found 21 days after application to alfalfa at a rate of 0.5 pounds/acre.

The chemical is quite toxic and in rats, the oral LD_{50} is 5.3 mg/kg, the percutaneous LD_{50} is 120 mg/kg and the toxic LD_{50} concentration for inhalation is 85 mg/m^3. In dogs, the oral LD_{50} is 19 mg/kg. The LD_{50} for ducks is 450 mcg/kg and for chickens is 6 mg/kg. Aquatic toxicity has shown that trout are sensitive at levels of 0.28 ppm after four days exposure.

The chemical is rapidly metabolized by mammals with over 90% excreted in the urine with a half-life of 6-12 hours. The principal metabolite is 3-hydroxy-furidan. Other metabolic breakdown products can also be identified. When given to cows, about 3% of the dose will be excreted in milk, mainly in the first 48 hours after exposure.

Like other carbamates, the chemical acts as a reversible cholinesterase inhibitor. In experimental animals given high, but nonlethal doses, cholinesterase returned to normal activity within four to six hours. When given in long-term experiments to rats, diets containing 25 ppm had no effect over two years, nor did 10 ppm have an effect over three generations. In dogs, diets containing 20 ppm had no effect over two years nor did 50 ppm have an effect over one generation. The principal route for toxicity is via ingestion or inhalation since the chemical is absorbed poorly through the skin.

In humans, toxicity is similar to other carbamates or organophosphates although the reaction is reversible and 2-PAM would be contraindicated in any illness. For specific therapy of intoxication see the section on medical treatment of carbamates at the end of this chapter. The chemical can be analyzed by either phosphorimetric means or by gas chromatography.

EPTC

EPTC, generically called S-ethyl dipropylthiocarbamate and also known under the names of Eptam, Stauffer R-1608 or Torbin, is a broadleaf herbicide. The molecular formula is $C_9H_{19}NOS$ and the structural formula is

$$C_2H_5S-CO-N(CH_2-CH_2-CH_3)_2$$

The molecular weight is 189.35 and the density is 0.955 at 30°C. The boiling point is 230°C and the flash point is 116°C. The chemical has a vapor pressure of 0.15 mm Hg. The chemical is soluble in water at 300-365 ppm. It is also miscible in a variety of organic solvents such as benzene, ethanol, toluene, xylene and acetone. It has an indefinite storage life under normal ambient conditions.

In experimental animals, the acute oral LD_{50} for rats is 1,630 mg/kg, the lowest effect for rats by inhalation is 200 mg/m^3/4 hours. In mice, the oral LD_{50} is 750 mg/kg. In cats, the oral LD_{50} is 112 mg/kg and the lower detectable effect via inhalation is 400 mg/m^3/4 hours. Birds are quite resistent to the effects of this chemical and the oral LC_{50} on quail is 26,000 ppm/7 days of the commercial formulation. Fish have a LC_{50} ranging from 17-21 ppm. In subacute feeding studies, rats fed a level of 16 mg/kg/day showed no effect in a 90 day study. Similarly, dogs showed no effect at 20 mg/kg/day. The chemical apparently is metabolized rapidly and after a 0.6 mg dose of Eptam given orally to rats, 8% was excreted in the urine, 4% in the feces, and 85% was excreted via the expired air. When the dosage was increased to approximately 100 mg, the amount excreted increased to 36%, 11% and 38% respectively for each route. Similarly, rats given varying dosages orally of radioactive

tagged EPTC had complete urinary elimination of the radio-
activity after 35 hours, for even the highest dosage.

In the environment, the chemical is rapidly broken
down by plants to carbon dioxide. There are other major
metabolites which can be found, including urea.

The chemical can be analyzed by spectrophotometric
method or by gas chromatography.

For specific therapy of intoxication see the section
on medical treatment of carbamates at the end of this
chapter.

The Ethylenebisdithiocarbamates

Chemical and Physical Properties

The accompanying table gives the common names for the
chemicals in this class. This also includes common tradenames which are registered.

Table 1.   EBDC Nomenclature

Common Name	Label Chemical Name	Tradename(s)
None	Diammonium EBDC	Amobam
Mancozeb	Mixture[1]	Dithane M-45
		Manzate 200
Maneb	Manganese EBDC	Manzate
		Dithane M-22
Nabam	Disodium EBDC	Parzate
		Dithane D-14
Metiram	Mixture[2]	Polyram
Zineb	Zinc EBDC	Dithane Z-78

[1]Mixture of zinc and manganese EBDC
[2]Mixture of ammoniates of EBDC

Table 2 represents chemical structure, molecular
formula, molecular weight, general physical properties
and solubility of the common EBDC's.

EBDC's are noted for their instability in the environment. They are easily degraded into a number of other
byproducts such as ethylene, ethylenebis-diisothiosulfide,
ethylenethiuram disulfide and ethylenethiuram monosulfide.
In particular, the application of heat will convert some
of these chemicals directly into ethylene and it is

Table 2.   Chemical and Physical Properties of EBDC's

Name	Molecular Formula	Molecular Weight	Physical Properties	Solubility
Amobam	$C_4H_{14}N_4S_4$	246.21	Unstable as dry material; aqueous solutions pale yellow to green; melting point 72.5° to 72.8°C	Soluble in water; slightly soluble in alcohol; insoluble in ben- and heptane
Mancozeb	Variable		Greyish-yellow powder which decomposes before melting; flash point 138°C	Practically insoluble in water and in most organic solvents
Maneb (monomer)	$C_4H_6N_2S_4Mn$	265.3	Yellow crystalline solid which decomposes before melting and on exposure to moisture or to acids	Slightly soluble in water and insoluble in most organic solvents

Table 2.(con't)   Chemical and Physical Properties of EBDC's

Name	Molecular Formula	Molecular Weight	Physical Properties	Solubility
Maneb (polymer)	$(C_4H_6MnN_2S_4)x$		Light-colored solid which decomposes before melting and on exposure to moisture or acids	Similar to monomer
Metiram	Indefinite		Light-yellow solid which melts above 120°C with decomposition; unstable under strongly acid or alkaline conditions or a combination of heat and moisture	Practically insoluble in water and in most organic solvents; soluble in decomposition in pyridine

ethylene residues which are commonly detected at levels
of 0.047 ppm to 0.083 ppm on spinach and oranges respectively. Thus the EBDC's can be broken down during the
process of cooking as well as by the natural process
occurring within the environment. It is believed that
breakdown of EBDC's to ethylenethiourea (ETU) from cooking of food ranges from 11 to 26% of the original compound.

Manufacturing Process

The chemicals are manufactured in a variety of formulations and methods. Briefly, Zineb is believed to occur
from a reaction of ethylenediamine (EDA) with carbon
disulfide (CS_2) in the presence of an alkali followed by
mixing Nabam with zinc sulfate. Maneb is prepared similarly to Zineb excepting that magnesium sulfate is used
in place of the zinc sulfate. Mancozeb is prepared from
an aqueous slurry of Maneb and a water soluble zinc salt.
Nabam and Amobam can also be manufactured from reactions
of EDA and CS_2, but in the presence of zinc oxide and
hydrogen peroxide, or by oxidation of an aqueous solution
of Nabam with hydrogen peroxide and subsequent precipita-
tion of zinc sulfate.

A number of formulations can then be made available
for commercial use in which the actual ingredients are in
the form of dust, wettable powders, solids, solutions or
suspensions of concentrates. Examples of such formulations are listed in Table 3.

The chemicals are registered for use on a variety of
food and field crops, particularly fruits and vegetables.
These chemicals may also be found in industrial circu-
lating water cooling towers, air washers, evaporating
condensers, pulp and paper mills, cane sugar mills,
leather, tobacco and ornamentals.

Teratogenicity

Kera (1973) studied ethylenethiourea (ETU) administration in rats in a variety of multiple doses and on a
daily basis. A teratogenic effect was seen at 10 mg/kg
and the no observable effect level (NOEL) was judged to
be 5 mg/kg. At the 10 mg/kg dosage, rats developed a
variety of neural crest defects, particularly menigo-
cephalocele, menigorrhagia, menigorrhea, hydrocephalus

Table 3. Formulations with EBDC's as sole active ingredients
All numbers are expressed as percentages

EBDC	Dust		Wet-table powders	Concentrates			Other
	Ready to use	Sprayed		Solid	Solution	Suspension	
Amobam					42-48		
Mancozeb	0.08-80	5.6-80	80	80	80		3.75 (fertilizer containing pesticide) 35 (granular pellets)
Maneb	1.4-50	80	40-90	40-80	37.42.5	25.80	1.9-10 (fertilizer containing pesticide) 1.4 (dust, pressurized) 3.2 (coating for inanimate surface)
Metiram	3.5-53.5		80	80			7 (nonaqueous solutions, used undiluted)
Nabam				22-93	22		22 (aqueous solution, used undiluted)
Zineb	5-19.5			75	75	25	6.5 (granular pellets)

and obliterated neural canal. In addition, some abnormal pelvic limb posture was seen as well as changes of the tail.

When given in a huge single oral dose (240 mg/kg), malformations also were induced which were again principally neural crest deformities although ectopic genitalia and nephrosis were also seen. Although the authors felt that the ETU was a unique teratogen in that it simultaneously produced malformations which they felt were mutually exclusive, (hydrocephalus and exencephaly), there are other teratogens which can induce the same type of defects, e.g. Vitamin A.

Carcinogenicity

Several oncogenic studies have been performed on individual chemicals as well as the principal breakdown product, ethylenethiourea (ETU).

Studies on Maneb in mice given a single weekly dose of 500 mg/kg body weight for a period of six weeks have been performed. In this case, lung adenomas developed in four of 42 test animals with none appearing in the control animals. In a different mice strain, lung adenomas developed in 23 of 42 test animals compared to 12 of 45 controls (Balin, 1970; IARC, 1976).

Zineb has been studied in mice of two strains in which they were given dosages of 3,500 mg/kg body weight by stomach tube for a period of six weeks. Lung adenomas were found in the treated animals of both strains and in the controls of strain "A" but not in the controls of the second strain. When the dosage of Zineb was decreased to 1,750 mg/kg body weight but given over a longer period of time (11 weeks), lung adenomas developed in the treated animals but not in the controls. In a review of the carcinogenicity of Zineb, the International Agency for Research on Cancer (IARC) concluded that Zineb does produce an increased incidence of lung tumors in mice.

The principal degradation product, ethylenethiourea (ETU) has been studied and found to be carcinogenic in both mice and rats. In mice, two strains of mice given a daily oral dose of ETU at 646 ppm daily for over 80 weeks developed liver tumors, lung tumors and lymphomas (Innes, 1969; National Cancer Institute, 1968). Liver tumors developed in 100% of both males and females treated in one strain and developed in 88% of the animals treated in the second strain.

In one strain of rats, ETU has been administered
orally in dosages of 175 and 350 ppm for 18 weeks.
Thyroid carcinomas were produced in test animals at
both dosages and did not occur in the controls. In
a second study, rats fed ETU in dosages ranging from
5-500 ppm for almost two years also developed thyroid
carcinomas at dosages of 250 and 500 ppm. Thyroid
adenomas developed at levels to 125 ppm, and, thyroid
hyperplasia developed at all dosages tested (Graham
1975). Thus, thyroid lesions were dose related with
the lower dosage producing hyperplasia and higher dosage
producing adenoma or carcinoma.

Human Toxicology

The principal experience with episodes of human intoxication or incidents has been with occupational exposure. The EPA's Pesticide Episode Response System
has reported only two episodes of EBDC problems from
the years 1972-1977. Both of these episodes involved
plane crashes in which aerial applicators were spraying
Mancozeb. No adverse effects upon humans, plants or
animals were reported in either of these two incidents.
Severe contact dermatitis has been reported in farm
workers who worked in fields sprayed with 0.5% suspension
of Zineb and who had repeated contact. The resulting
dermatitis was generally extensive and severe (Zorin,
1970).

Medical Treatment of Carbamates

Carbamates, as a class, inhibit cholinesterase. The
routes of absorption may be either by ingestion, inhalation or via the dermal route. The general lack of solubility in lipids makes them less toxic via the dermal
route than by other methods. Cholinesterase inhibition
is reversible and delayed neuropathy does not occur.

Symptoms

In general, symptoms of carbamate intoxication are
very similar to that of the organophosphates, however,
the length and severity of such symptoms are generally
not as severe as with the organophosphates and treatment

is generally simpler. Early symptoms would include
excessive salivation or sweating and a sense of fatigue
or weakness. Constriction of pupils will occur in severe
intoxication. Muscle incoordination, as the result of
prolonged muscle fibrillation or muscle twitching, can
be seen. Nausea, vomiting and diarrhea will occur along
with abdominal cramps if intoxication is severe enough
and complaints of some sense of tightness in the chest
or dyspnea may occur as the result of restriction of the
intercostal muscles.

First Aid

It is important that the chemical be removed as quickly as possible. In the case of skin contact, the area
should be washed carefully with soap and water. It is
generally preferred for the person administering first
aid to wear some protection such as rubber gloves while
washing the contact area. In massive overdose, it is
again important to recall that acute respiratory failure
may occur as the result of paralysis of the respiratory
muscles.

Specific Treatment

In mild cases of carbamate intoxication it has been
noted that the symptoms may be reversed very simply by
any alkaloid, even tincture of belladonna. In more
severe cases, specific treatment is the use of atropine
intramuscularly or intravenously in dosages of 2-4 mg
given every 10-15 minutes until signs of atropinization
or complete reversal of symptoms occur. It is important
to keep the airway open and to prevent aspiration if
nausea and vomiting is a problem. In the case of ingestion, lavage can be performed followed by the ingestion of 5% sodium bicarbonate. The use of 2-PAM is
contraindicated! Atropine is the drug of choice. The
patient should be observed carefully during the early
stages of treatment, again the principal concern being
that of respiratory arrest. Certain drugs such as theo-
phylline, aminophylline or barbiturates are to be avoided.

Diagnostic Studies

Serum or plasma should be analyzed immediately for
cholinesterase levels to confirm the diagnosis of carbamate intoxication. Urine is not measured for carbamate
directly, however, 1-napthol, which is normally found in
trace amounts in urine, is found in much higher concentrations following carbaryl (Sevin) ingestion and may be
looked for in this specific instance only.

References

Balin, P.N. (1970) Experimental data on the blastomo-
    genic activity of the fungicide Maneb. Vrach Delo
    4:21-24.

Blevins, R.D., W. Lijinsky and J.D. Regan (1977) Nitro-
    sated methylcarbamate insecticides: Effect on the DNA
    of human cells. Mutat Res 44:1-7.

Fukuto, T.R. (1972) Metabolism of carbamate insecticides.
    Drug Metab Revs 1:117-151.

Graham, S.L.K. (1975) Effects of prolonged ethylenethio-
    urea ingestion on the thyroid of the rat. Food Cosmet
    Toxicol 113:493-499.

Innes, J.R.M. (1969) Bioassay of pesticides and indus-
    trial chemicals for tumorigenicity in mice: A pre-
    liminary note. J Nat Cancer Inst 42:1101-1114.

International Agency for Research on Cancer (1976)   IARC
    monograph on the evaluation of carcinogenic risk of
    chemicals to man. Lyon, France. 12:137-149.

Khera, K.S. (1973) Ethylenethiourea teratogenicity
    study in rats and rabbits. Teratology 7:243-252.

Morbidity and Mortality Weekly Report (1979) Suspected
    carbamate intoxication - Nebraska. 28:133-134.

National Cancer Institute (1968) Evaluation of carcino-
    genic, teratogenic and mutagenic activities of select-
    ed pesticides and industrial chemicals. Carcinogenic
    Study, National Technical Information Service, U.S.
    Department of Commerce, Washington, DC. 1:61-62.

Schlinke, J.C. (1977) Toxicologic effects of five soil
  nematocides in cattle and sheep. Amer J Vet Res
  31:1364-1366.

Seiler, J.P. (1977) Nitrosation in vitro and in vivo
  by sodium nitrite and mutagenicity of nitrogenous
  pesticides. Mutat Res 48:225-236.

Woodham, D.W., R.G. Reeves and R.R. Edwards (1973)
  Total toxic aldicarb residues in weeds, grasses,
  and wildlife from the Texas high plains following
  a soil treatment with insecticides. J Agric Food
  Chem 21:604-607.

Zorin, P.M. (1970) Allergic dermatitis developing as
  a result of contact with Zineb. Vestn Dermatol
  Venerol 44:65-68.

6

Halogenated Hydrocarbons
and Organotins

Dicofol

Dicofol is a chemical of the chlorinated hydrocarbon class with a molecular formula of $C_{14}H_9Cl_5O$ and the structural formula is as follows:

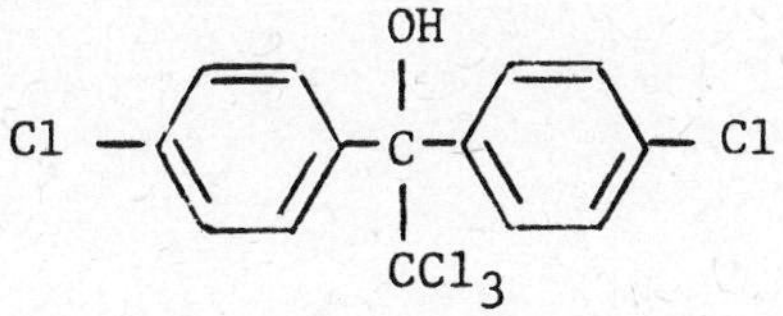

The chemical's generic name is 1,1-bis(p-chloro-phenyl)-2,2,2-trichloroethanol. It is marketed under the tradenames Kelthane, Acarin and Mitigan.

The chemical has a molecular weight of 370.5. The pure compound is a white solid with a melting point of 79°C, however, the technical product is a light brown viscous oil with a density of 1.45. The chemical is insoluble in water but soluble in most aliphatic and aromatic products and is lipophilic. The chemical is hydrolyzed by alkali to dichlorobenzophenone and chloroform.

The chemical is manufactured by the chlorination of bis(4-chlorophenyl) carbinol. Its principal use in agriculture is as an acaricide and in the Pacific Northwest it is used particularly on grain crops such as alfalfa and hops. It is also registered for use on vegetables, fruits and a variety of field crops and is

used widely in nurseries and greenhouses. The chemical
is relatively stable although when heated, or in contact
with strong acids, it decomposes to evolve toxic hydrogen
chloride fumes. The chemical is also produced by the
detoxification of DDT.

The chemical is believed to be fairly stable in the
environment and after application, although residues
decrease rapidly, traces can be found in soil a year
later.

In experimental animals, the acute oral LD_{50} for rats
is 809 mg/kg (males) and 684 mg/kg (females). In chronic
feeding experiments, dogs fed one year on a diet containing 300 ppm showed no evidence of histopathological
changes. Rats fed a diet containing 1,000 ppm for two
years showed no changes in weight, however, rats fed a
diet for two years at levels of 250 ppm or higher showed
depression of growth and skin changes of erythema and
superficial necrosis. At high levels, animals show
symptoms compatible with chlorinated hydrocarbon intoxication, namely, central nervous system effects and
renal and kidney changes. The chemical also is fairly
irritating when animals are treated subcutaneously or
dermally with signs of contact dermatitis.

In humans, dermatitis may be predicted but experience
has shown that it occurs only rarely. There are no
reported cases of systemic intoxication from Kelthane.
Laboratory methods allow for the analysis of this chemical via a number of systems but principally flame photo-
metry or colorimetry. The preferred method may be gas
chromatography. In mammals, the chemical may be broken
down to dichlorobenzophenone or dichlorobenzohydrol and
these may be the products which need to be monitored.

Plictran

Plictran is a chemical which has the generic name
tricyclohexylhydroxystannane. It is also marketed under
the name Plyctran, Cyhexatin and Dowco 213.

The chemical has a molecular formula of $C_{18}H_{34}OSn$.
The structural formula is as follows:

It is used mainly as an acaricide.

The chemical has a melting point of 195-198°C. It has a negligible weight vapor pressure of 25°C. It exists as a white crystal and is fairly stable in both neutral and alkaline suspensions. It is degraded by ultraviolet light.

The chemical is only slightly soluble in water, less than 1 ppm at 25°C. It is very soluble in chloroform and in methanol.

In experimental animals the acute oral LD_{50} for rats is 540 mg/kg; for guinea pigs, 780 mg/kg; and for chickens 654 mg/kg. Chronic feeding experiments with rats fed 16 weeks on a diet containing 200 ppm showed reduced weight gain apparently because of unpalatability of the diet. Similarly, dogs fed 12 months on a diet containing 12 ppm showed nutritional deficiencies. Since rats do not readily accept a diet containing this chemical, in one investigation, 25 mg/kg/day was fed by single dose gavage over a period of two weeks. At this level of treatment, there were microscopic changes found in the liver, kidney and the adrenal glands. In beagle dogs, 3 mg/kg/day was felt to be a no effect level based upon body weight gain. In dogs fed 6 mg/kg/day for two years, there was evidence of slower growth rate but there were no apparent toxicological or pathological changes. Rats on long-term feeding experiments of 12 mg/kg/day for two years showed no evidence of changes either grossly or by histopathological examination after two years. A level of 6 mg/kg/day is now considered the no effect level for rats. In this study, there were no effects on fertility, gestation, viability or lactation observed in the rats over three generations. In teratology studies, female rabbits who received oral doses of 3 mg/kg day on the sixth through the 16th day of gestation showed no evidence of abnormalities.

There are no reported cases of systemic intoxication from this chemical. Analytical methods for determining organotins can be performed by titration potentiometrically with perchloric acid or via colorimetric methods.

7

Substituted Ureas

Diuron

Diuron, generically called 3-(3,4-dichlorophenyl)-1,1-
dimethylurea, is also known as Karmex, Diurex, Vonduron,
DMU, Herbatox and Dailon. It is a chemical with a molecular formula of $C_{19}H_{10}Cl_2N_2O$ and the structural formula
is as follows:

$$Cl - \text{(ring, Cl)} - NH.C.N(CH_3)_2 \quad (O)$$

It finds its major use as a pre-emergence herbicide on
a variety of field crops and is also used on fruit and
vegetable crops.

The chemical has a molecular weight of 233.10 and a
melting point of 158-159°C. Vapor pressure is low at
3.1×10^{-6} mm Hg at 50°C. It is an odorless, white crystalline solid in the pure form and is stable to oxidation
and moisture. It does hydrolyze easily in fairly strong
acids or alkali. It is non-corrosive under usual shelf
conditions. It is only slightly soluble in water at
42 ppm at 25°C and has a very low solubility in hydrocarbons. In acetone, it is soluble at 5.3% at 27°C. It
is decomposed at 190°C. A variety of formulatons exist
on the market which may contain mixtures of different
herbicides. For example, Diurol is a mixture of 50%
diuron and 30% amitrol. Krovar-I contains 40% diuron
and 40% bromacil.

In experimental animals, the acute oral LD_{50} for rats is 3400 mg/kg. Its limits of aquatic toxicity to fish are apparently about 1-10 ppm/96 hours of exposure. In birds, mallards have an LD_{50} of above 2,000 mg/kg. Two year feeding studies in which rats were administered diuron at rates of 174-464 mg/kg/day found no evidence of carcinogenesis after two years. On the other hand, rats and dogs fed high levels of diuron via the diet showed evidence of anemia, retarded growth, hyperspleno-megaly, hepatomegaly, and splenic hemosiderosis at levels of 2500 ppm. It is also conceivable that prolonged exposure at high levels might be responsible for bone marrow changes.

Metabolism in mammals has been studied and in rats, the compound is broken down principally to N-(3,4-di-chlorophenyl)urea. Methyl urea metabolite and 3,4-di-chloroaniline are also present along with dichlorophenol. Excretion of metabolites is mainly in the urine but may also be found in feces. The production of the dichloro-aniline breakdown product may be responsible for the formation of methemoglobinemia in animals.

In humans poisoned by diuron, dimethyl and methyl urea compound were isolated from the urine along with dichloroaniline.

The compound is quite stable in the environment and may persist in soil for several years at an effective level. It is extremely resistent to attack by micro-organisms and estimates of the half-life at 20°C have been in the order of ten years.

In humans, the expected effects would first be those of primary irritation of the mucous membranes of the eye, ear, nose and throat as well as the skin. Central nervous system depression along with respiratory de-pression may occur leading to a secondary hypoxemia. The liberation of the p-chloroanaline may lead to a methemoglobinemia which requires specific treatment.

Initial treatment of humans would be to prevent ab-sorption, therefore, skin or mucous membranes should be flushed with tap water or saline. Activated charcoal at 5-10 times estimated dosage should be given in a water slurry orally or by lavage and repeated at least one time.

Methemoglobin levels should be immediately checked for and methylene blue should be available in case evid-ence of methemoglobinemia occurs. If central nervous system signs occur, diazapam may be given in dosages of 10 mg in adults or 0.10-0.30 mg/kg in children. Patients should be followed carefully for respiratory depression, including the possible necessity for endotrachial intubation.

Laboratory analysis of urine or stool can be performed using methods of gas chromatography or thin layer chromatography.

Linuron

Linuron has the generic name of 3-(3,4-dichlorophenyl)-1-methoxy-1-methylurea. It is a substituted urea herbicide and commonly known under the name of Lorox. Other alternative names are Afalon, Sinuron, Premalin and Sarclex.

The chemical is used for the control of broadleaf weeds particularly in vegetable and grain crops. In the Pacific Northwest it is used principally on wheat.

The chemical has a molecular weight of 249.11 and a melting point of 93-94°C. In the pure form it is an odorless white crystalline solid. It is non-corrosive and stable in solution. It is only slightly soluble in water at 275 ppm but is quite soluble in acetone, benzene, ethanol and xylene.

Its toxicity in experimental animals reveals an acute oral LD_{50} in rats of 1500 mg/kg and in dogs of 500 mg/kg. It is a mild irritant in skin tests with guinea pigs when applied as a 50% suspension. Chronic feeding experiments of linuron to rats and dogs for two years at dietary levels of 2500 ppm have been performed with a breakdown product of aniline residues found in the blood and fat, liver, kidney and spleen. It is believed to be of low toxicity with chronic exposure. When given to rats in dosages of 200 mg/kg for 10 days, while weight gain was depressed, there was no evidence of histopathological changes, however, high dosages have shown hemolytic effects with increased erythropoeisis. Carcinogenicity studies performed in rats and dogs showed no tumors and rabbits fed doses of 25-125 ppm during the eighth to 16th day of pregnancy showed no embryotoxic or teratogenic effects.

Metabolism studies in rats have demonstrated that the chemical is metabolized into 3,4-dichloroaniline plus a variety of dichlorophenyl ureas, methyl urea and dichlorophenols. It is then excreted as a glucuronide or sulfate.

In the environment, the chemical is broken down principally by microbial action with the breakdown products

consisting of 3,4-dichloroaniline and carbon dioxide.
The chemical is adsorbed on soil or organic matter and
does not move freely. The chemical is not believed to
accumulate with annual application although phytotoxic
concentrations may be present for as long as four months.

There are no reported cases of intoxication from
linuron, however, concern would be in the hematopoetic
system followed by hepatic changes.

In examining for possible exposure, analysis of urine
would be performed for breakdown products. In addition,
the blood should be screened for evidence of either
compensated or noncompensated hemolytic anemia.

8

Nitrophenols

Dinoseb

Dinoseb, generically called 2-sec-butyl-4,6-dinitro-phenol, is also known under the names of Chemox, Buta-phene, Premerge, DNBP and Knoxweed. The molecular formula is $C_{10}H_{12}O_5N_2$ and the structural formula is as follows:

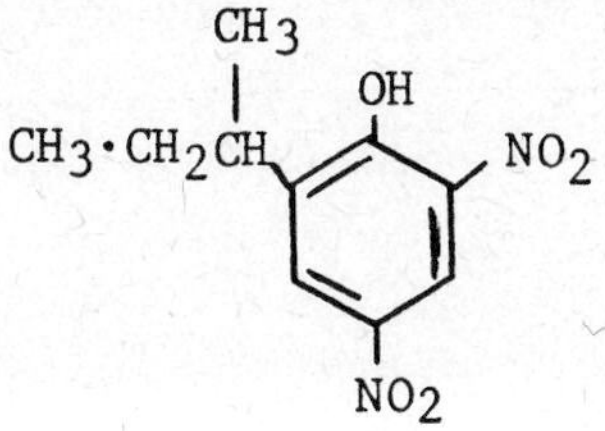

$$CH_3 \cdot CH_2CH \underset{\overset{|}{CH_3}}{} \begin{array}{c} OH \\ \end{array} NO_2$$

NO_2

The chemical is used principally as an herbicide.
Dinoseb has a melting point of 42°C. The molecular weight is 192.94. It is only slightly soluble in water although a variety of soluble salts can be marketed. The chemical is freely soluble in a number of organic sol-vents, oils and ethanol. The chemical is moderately corrosive and when shipped or stored should be kept in a cool place since it has potential for breaking down and as a fire hazard. In the latter case, there is the potential for nitrate formation.
Dinoseb is considered to be a very toxic herbicide. In rats, the oral LD_{50} is 26 mg/kg and the percutaneous

LD_{50} is 80 mg/kg. In mice, the oral LD_{50} is 20 mg/kg.
In guinea pigs, the oral LD_{50} is 20 mg/kg but the percutaneous LD_{50} is 500 mg/kg. The parent compound is
metabolized by being enzymatically reduced in the liver
to a variety of primary amines. Studies demonstrate
that following exposure the chemical is found principally
in the liver, kidney, spleen and the blood. In the
urine, both the unchanged compound and the metabolites
can be found. In chronic feeding experiments with ducks,
cataracts were found with a diet containing 50 ppm. In
rats, diets containing 100 ppm fed for six months produced no ill effects.

In humans, symptoms can be expected to be similar to
those of other nitrophenols. In particular, the chemical
acts by being an uncoupler of oxidative phosphorylation
and the syndrome occurring is secondary to that phenomenon. The chemical also is a skin irritant and will cause
a contact dermatitis.

Laboratroy methods for analysis include thin layer
chromatography, spectrophotometry and polarography.

Human Experience With Nitrophenols

The experience of human intoxication with the nitrophenol herbicides has been reviewed and summarized by
Bidstrup and co-workers (1951, 1952) in several articles.
In the reviews, Bidstrup was principally concerned with
the herbicide dinitro-ortho-cresol but also was cognizant
of dinitrophenols. Interestingly, the latter was used
for a period of time in the 1930's as a method of treating obesity, the reasoning being that the chemical caused
a hypermetabolic rate. The practice was discontinued
because of either accidental overdosage, development of
agranulocytosis or the development of cataracts.

Early symptoms and signs include fatigue, insomnia,
sweating, thirst, weight loss and headache. By the time
such symptoms occur, the individual is well along on the
way to intoxication and Bidstrup suggested (1952) that a
premonitory subjective symptom may be a sensation of
euphoria. Yellow discoloration of the sclera may occur
and indicates absorption of the chemical rather than the
development of jaundice. Similarly, the skin may be
stained yellow as a result of the chemical although skin
discoloration represents exposure, but not necessarily
an excessive amount.

The blood and urine may be monitored. It is clear
that the whole blood is a better indicator than urine.
Bidstrup recommended, in the case of DNOC, that a level
of 20 mcg/g of blood would indicate a time to remove a
person from work. Blood levels of 40 mcg/g of blood,
would be associated with toxic symptoms. Such a low
safety margin would undoubtedly not be considered acceptable today. Interestingly, at levels of 20 mcg/g of
blood, further exposure led to marked increases in the
blood levels suggesting that a maximum threshold of
excretion exists in humans, beyond which the chemical
will accumulate rapidly. Following exposure, the blood
levels have demonstrated detectable amounts lasting for
more than 40 days. In suspected cases of intoxication,
treatment should not be delayed while awaiting laboratory
confirmation. The similarity to acute hyperthyroidism
or a thyroid crisis can be utilized as a means of following, as well as confirming, suspicions. It has been
demonstrated that the basal metabolic rate (BMR) will be
strikingly elevated under conditions of nitrophenol intoxication and it is anticipated that thyroid hormones
such as T-3 and T-4 would be normal. The BMR can probably be used as a means of simple and long-term follow-up.

Medical Treatment

The treatment of nitrophenols is initially directed
at the prevention of absorption. Thus, contaminated
clothing should be removed and the skin washed with soap
and water. If the patient has ingested the chemical,
and is alert, Syrup of Ipecac may be used. If the patient
is not fully conscious, then intubation should be performed and the stomach lavaged with saline. Activated
charcoal should either be swallowed or administered via
the gastric tube and a saline cathartic to promote rapid
excretion is advisable.
    In the event that intoxication is severe, central
nervous system excitation does occur and should be treated
symptomatically with an agent such as diazapam or with a
barbiturate. Antipyretic medications, such as aspirin,
are contraindicated since aspirin may react synergistically with nitrophenol to increase, rather than to improve,
the problem. Other chemicals which might normally be
considered useful in this situation, such as atropine,
should also not be used.

During the acute phase, attempts should be made to reduce body temperature and decrease the metabolic rate such as with the use of cooling blankets or alcohol sponging.

The patient should be followed with serial analyses of the urine for levels of the chemical and convalescence may be delayed because of a relatively slow release from the body.

References

Bidstrup, P.L. and D.J.H. Payne (1951) Poisoning by dinitro-ortho-cresol. Br Med J 2:16-19.

Bidstrup, P.L, J.A.L. Bonnell and D.G. Harvey (1952) Prevention of acute dinitro-ortho-cresol (DNOC) poisoning. Lancet 262:794-795.

9

Fungicides

The use of chemical fungicides is frequently not considered a major environmental concern by members of the public although the general class of chemicals have now raised certain questions regarding their long-term safety, particularly in regard to possible biodegradation to potential carcinogens. The latter statement is particularly true of the carbamate fungicides. From the economic standpoint, if chemical fungicides were not available, certain crop losses might be as high as 100%, as in the use on grapes, or, 75% for peanuts. Other examples could be cited.

The loss estimates have been stated in an official report, "Fungicides: An Overview of Their Significance to Agriculture and Their Regulatory Implications" by the Economic Analysis Branch and Plant Sciences Branch, Benefits and Field Studies Division, OPP, EPA. The fungicides of interest were mainly those based on the ethylenebisdithiocarbamates, captan, benomyl, pentachloronitrobenzene, DBCP and soil fumigants. This report estimated that 145 million pounds of fungicides were produced in 1974 and also estimated that without fungicide treatment of seeds, 25% of the wheat and oat crops would be lost. Thus, the use of these chemicals has a significant impact on agricultural production.

Copper Sulfate

Copper sulfate is generically $CuSO_4 \cdot 5H_2O$. The chemical is known either by its generic name or is commonly

279

referred to as Bluestone. It may also be seen under the name of Vitriol. In the Pacific Northwest it is used as a fungicide on fruit crops such as apples and pears. The chemical has a variety of other uses in industry such as in petroleum refining, as a pigment in paints, in adhesives, in anti-rusting compositions and in photo engraving.

It has a molecular weight of 249.68. At $110^{\circ}C$, four molecules of water are lost and at $150^{\circ}C$, the boiling point is reached and the remaining water is lost. The density is 2.286. At $650^{\circ}C$, the compound decomposes to form copper II oxide (CuO). It is a blue crystalline compound which is very soluble in water at rates of 31.6 g/100 cc water at $0^{\circ}C$ and 203.3 g/100 cc at $100^{\circ}C$. It is also slightly soluble in methanol, glycerol and ethanol.

In experimental animals, toxicity experiments show an acute oral LD_{50} in rats of 300 mg/kg. In guinea pigs, the subcutaneous no observable effect level is 62 mg/kg. In bass, an LD_{50} occurs of 1 ppm after 96 hours exposure. Long-term feeding experiments in rats at levels of 500 ppm have caused retarded growth and at 4,000 ppm have caused death. In pigs fed a diet containing 0.1% of copper sulfate for a long term, skin changes developed consisting mainly of parakeratosis and eczematous-like changes.

Considerable experience has been gained with this chemical in veterinary medicine where acute intoxication episodes have occurred with findings principally related to acute hepatic necrosis although there has also been evidence of hemolytic anemia and abdominal complaints with a generalized gastroenteritis. The chemical also appears to be a primary respiratory irritant in animals.

Because the chemical is commonly used in treatment of water to control algae growth, studies have been performed relating to the toxicity to fish and levels somewhere in the area of 1-5 ppm are considered to be in a potentially toxic range.

In humans, the chemical can be analyzed for directly either in the blood or in the urine.

Pentachloronitrobenzene

Pentachloronitrobenzene is a commonly used fungicide frequently marketed under the names of Quintozene, Penta- gen, Folosan and Terrachlor, among others. The chemical has a molecular formula of $C_6Cl_5NO_2$ and the structural formula is as follows:

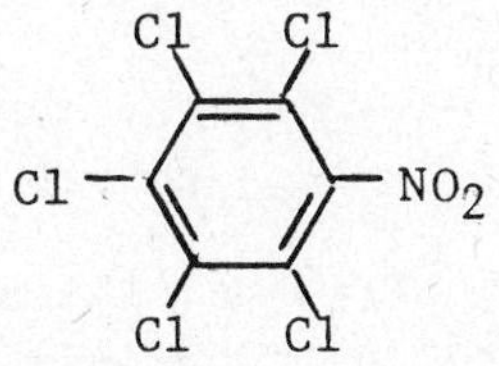

The chemical has a molecular weight of 295.32 and a density of 1.718 at 25°C. It has low volatility with a vapor pressure of 133×10^{-4} mm Hg. It is a crystalline solid and is stable and non-corrosive. It is insoluble in water but is freely soluble in organic solvents such as benzene, chloroform and carbon disulfide. The melting point of the technical product is 142-145°C and the boiling point is 328°C.

In experimental animals, the chemical has an oral LD_{50} in rats of 1650 mg/kg and in mice of 2500 mg/kg. It is also a demonstrated teratogen and carcinogen in mice at 2500 mg/kg and 135 mg/kg respectively.

It is usually manufactured as a wettable powder or as an emulsifiable concentrate. It has been approved in the United States for use as a soil fungicide on ornamental crops and as a treatment on certain grain seeds.

Hexachlorobenzene may be present as an impurity in the technical product.

After applications of large amounts, such as 25 pounds per acre, the chemical has been found at levels of 0.1 ppm in food products.

In soils, the chemical is converted to pentachloro-aniline.

In experimental animals, long-term feeding studies in rats of up to 500 ppm and in beagle dogs of up to 1,080 ppm, demonstrated no PCNB present in the tissues although pentachloroaniline was detected in small amounts. Administration of the chemical to rabbits showed that 62% was excreted unchanged in the feces and the remainder was excreted either as pentachloroaniline or as a pentachloro-phenylcystine. The chemical is poorly absorbed in mammals and is mainly excreted through the feces.

In long-term studies, mice fed 464 mg/kg by stomach tube beginning at seven days of age until 28 days of age and then transferred to a diet containing 1,206 ppm up to the age of 78 weeks, developed hepatomas. Similarly,

chronic feeding studies of three months in rats fed
5,000 ppm in their diet were performed and at autopsy
livers were enlarged and showed some vacuolization of
cytoplasm. In contrast, rats have survived two year
feeding tests at dietary levels of 2500 ppm, apparently
without ill effects.

The chemical is considered a carcinogen by current
NIOSH standards.

In humans, the chemical is believed to be a skin
irritant and sensitizer leading to contact dermatitis.
Because of the possibility of hexachlorobenzene contamination, consideration should be given to the development of porphyria cutanea tarda in people who ingest
very large dosages for a lengthy period of time. Because of the hepatotoxic effect, the administration of
other hepatotoxic drugs might be expected to be synergistic.

Laboratory analysis is performed by gas chromatography.

Karathane

Karathane is a fungicide and acaricide which is used
in the Pacific Northwest in the treatment of fruit,
mainly pears and apples. The molecular formula is
$C_{18}H_{24}N_2O_6$ and the structural formula is as follows:

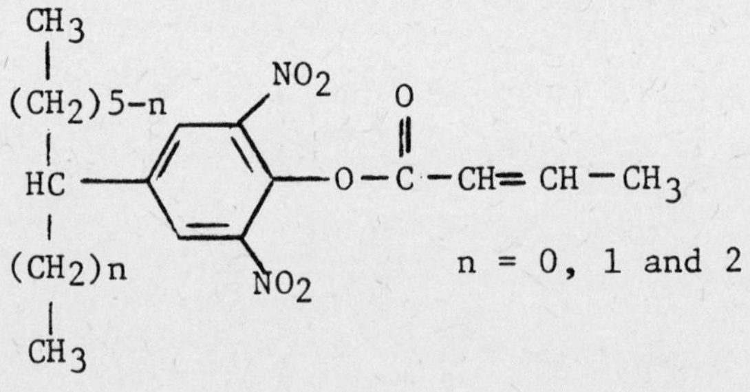

The chemical generically is 2,4-dinitro-6-octylphenyl
crotonate. It is a crotonic acid and is marketed under
a variety of other names such as Arathane, Mildex, Iso-
cothan and Dinocap. It has a molecular weight of 364.44;
a boiling point of 138-148°C. It is a dark brown liquid
which is insoluble in water but soluble in organic chemicals such as chloroform and petrochemicals such as
benzene and ether. Commercial formulations are commonly
as a dust or powder or as an emulsifiable concentrate.

In experimental animals, the compound has an acute LD_{50} in rats of 980 mg/kg. Long-term feeding experiments in dogs fed 50 ppm in the diet for one year produced no ill effects. Ducks fed 50 ppm developed cataracts.

In human beings, there are no reported cases of systemic intoxication, however, the chemical should be expected to react like a dinitrophenol. It can easily be absorbed through the skin. It is an irritant that will produce both a conjunctivitis and irritation of the mucous membranes, especially of the upper airway. In addition, it might produce a hyper metabolic state with fever, increased sweating and thirst. With prolonged or increased exposure, gastrointestinal, hepatic and central nervous system signs would appear.

Routine clinical laboratory studies would be likely to show hepatic enzyme changes, leukopenia, possibly changes suggesting a nephropathy and also a neuropathy.

Residues of the chemical should be analyzable by a variety of spectrophotometric methods and it would be expected that residue should be found in the urine and blood.

10

Fumigants

Agricultural chemicals in the fumigant class are used
in a number of different situations. Chemicals are used
both prior to planting and post harvest. This class of
chemicals has been utilized in agriculture for many years
and is among the oldest of the known insecticides. Methyl
bromide, which will be discussed in detail, can be used
as an example. This chemical is used in soil as a means
of killing soil nematodes. Under some circumstances,
soil fumigation with methyl bromide will triple the crop
of fruits such as strawberries. Following harvest,
methyl bromide may be used as a fumigant on stored grain,
a common means of preventing a variety of insects or worms
from destroying the stored crop. In seaports, crops of a
number of different types can be inspected prior to their
being removed from a ship's hold. If insects are noted,
the holds are immediately closed and fumigated with methyl
bromide. This has been found effective in preventing
transportation of insects into this country - an improvement in both the environment and public health.
Although a number of fumigants are in use, methyl
bromide will be used as an example of a common one and
its toxicology discussed in more detail.

Methyl Bromide

Methyl bromide, with a structural formula of CH3Br, is
also known as a bromomethane and known under the tradenames of Metafume or Metabrom. The chemical has a molecular weight of 94.95. It is a colorless and odorless

284

gas excepting in very high concentrations when it has a
sweetish, chloroform-like odor. It has a boiling point
of only 4.5°C and a freezing point of -93°C. Its vapor
pressure at 20°C is 1120 mm Hg. The specific gravity of
the liquid is 1.732 and that of the vapor is 3.974 (air
equal to one). It is soluble in most organic solvents,
however, in aqueous solution, it is slowly hydrolyzed
with the formation of methanol and hydrobromic acid. The
mixture of methanol and hydrobromic acid is also the
starting point in the manufacture of the chemical in
which the two are reacted and then separated by distillation.

Animal Toxicity: The toxicity of methyl bromide has
been reviewed by van Oettingen (1964). Because the chemical is a gas under normal conditions, the expression of
toxicity is via inhalation and frequently includes a time
factor. For example, mice exposed to concentrations of
methyl bromide of 500-600 ppm showed no fatalities at a
duration of 90 minutes. When the duration of exposure
was increased to 180 minutes, all animals died. The LD_{50},
therefore, is not readily interpretable, although in rats,
it has been set at 20 mg/l (approximately 5100 ppm). The
chemical is toxic in man as well. The toxic effects are
frequently delayed and do not appear for a number of
hours after cessation of exposure. In man, a safe upper
limit has been set at 17 ppm, above which concentration
respirators are to be worn. Under conditions of exposure
experimental animals show evidence of pulmonary hemorrhage, acute kidney injury and central nervous system
signs including paralysis, weakness, coma and convulsions.
It is interesting that acute exposures may be associated
with no ill effects upon animals, even though the exposure may be at fairly high concentrations. On the other
hand, repeated exposure to methyl bromide in small concentrations may lead to the development of pathological
symptoms and signs. The biological half-life in blood
is about 11 hours.
     The mechanism of toxic action is not completely under-
stood. It is believed that the chemical passes through
the cellular membrane with some difficulty which partly
explains its prolonged or delayed action. In the cell,
the chemical appears to react with sulfhydryl groups,
inactivating a number of enzyme systems that are dependent upon the availability of the sulfhydryl system.
     The chemical is not known to be mutagenic, carcino-
genic or teratogenic.

Human Toxicology: Because the inorganic bromide
salts, such as sodium bromide, were used extensively
in the treatment of epilepsy prior to the discovery of
phenytoin, considerable experience with the bromide ion
as such developed during the early part of this century.
A complete review on bromide intoxication was published
by Moore, Sohler and Alexander (1940). The symptoms of
bromide intoxication with the inorganic bromides are very
similar to those of the organic compounds, such as methyl
bromide, with the exception that there is a predominance
of central nervous system signs with the organic bromides.
   Bromides are widely distributed through the body.
There seems to be a predilection for bromide to concentrate in the central nervous system. The latter was
suggested to be a type of "sink" by Pollay (1967).
Bromide may also appear, perhaps somewhat unexpectedly,
in the gastric mucosa and, therefore, in the gastric
secretions. The gastric contents could be a means of
determining bromide excess in the human, although other
means are simpler. The chemical is secreted selectively
via the kidneys with bromide having a preferential route
of excretion over chlorides. Forced renal excretion is
the principal method of treatment of bromide intoxication.
Bromides have also been associated with hypercholesterol-
emia by Rosenblum and associates (1963).
   The biological half-life of bromide in blood varies
with the mammal studied. In experimental animals such
as mice, the biological half-life was found to be 1.5
days. On the other hand, in human beings, the biological
half-life in blood has been found to be 12 days. This
very extended half-life accounts in part for the toxicity
seen with prolonged exposure in small dosages, since the
steady state is reached many days after the initial
exposure and repeated exposures of what would normally
be considered innocuous levels can, therefore, lead to
high levels in the blood. On the other hand, the lengthy
biological half-life has been utilized in the application
of the inorganic bromide as an aneleptic because it
allowed for a constant concentration in the blood and
careful control of epilepsy.

First Aid For Exposure: Exposure to methyl bromide
will usually occur via the respiratory or dermal route.
It is important to remove clothing immediately in order
to prevent it from being absorbed, following which, the
skin can be washed with soap and water. In the event of
inadvertant respiratory exposure, the patient can only

be removed from the contaminated environment. In working
conditions, however, it is important to know whether
bromide is present in the air, since workers should not
be exposed to repeated concentrations, even at low levels.

   Symptoms and Signs of Intoxication: Illness from
methyl bromide must be separated into the acute versus
the chronic syndromes. The acute effects are principally
related to marked irritation of the eyes, the skin and
the mucous membranes, including the upper and lower
respiratory tract. The chemical is quite irritating to
the skin and will not only produce a fairly severe contact dermatitis, but in some cases, will lead to secondary burns with the formation of vesicles and bullae.
The chemical is usually absorbed on clothing which must
be removed quickly to prevent further skin contact.
The acute effects also include considerable irritation
of the eyes with tearing and development of conjunctivitis
as well as irritation of the nasal membranes. In high
concentrations, methyl bromide may cause enough lung
irritation to produce pulmonary edema. Acute exposure
may lead to central nervous system depression with malaise, headaches, somnolence, vertigo and tremor. In
addition, visual disturbances may develop as well as
nausea and vomiting. Epileptiform seizures have been
reported although the depression of the central nervous
system generally occurs in a gradual, but progressive
form. It is critical to note that symptoms may frequently
be delayed considerably from the exposure time to the
onset of symptoms. The delay is usually from 30 minutes
to six hours but may allegedly occur as late as 48 hours.
Therefore, any patient with bona fide exposure to methyl
bromide should be observed for this period of time and
possibly even treatment begun in order to prevent the
delayed syndrome.
   With chronic exposure, as may occur with low grade
repeated exposures from fumigants or from inhaling methyl
bromide which has been inappropriately stored, the symptoms appear almost entirely in the central nervous system
with changes of mental confusion, lethargy, difficulty
with vision, such as focusing, decreased concentration
and so forth.

   Diagnostic Studies: There is no specific test that
can be utilized for methyl bromide as such, however, the
serum bromide is frequently used as a means of confirming suspected intoxication. The test is not very good .

for the performance of routine monitoring of workers.
It is important to confer with the clinical pathologist
to determine exactly what method of bromide measurement
is performed since a variety of methods are available
which differ in what might be considered normal. Although with inorganic bromides, toxicity is not generally
considered until the serum level is greater than 50 mg%,
the same is not true for methyl bromide. Case reports
of chronic intoxication exist in which levels are less
than 10 mg%, although these levels would normally be
considered well within normal range and quite safe for
inorganic bromide. In general, it is believed that the
spinal fluid concentration would be approximately two-
thirds that of the blood serum.

Methyl Bromide - Clinical Symptoms and Signs

An excellent review of seven cases of methyl bromide
intoxication reported by Rathus and Landy (1961) demonstrates the importance of serial blood bromide levels and
the need to perform the tests by an accurate method.
Symptoms in this series are almost entirely related to
central nervous system intoxication with complete recovery noted, even though the exposure was severe. The
importance of appropriate respiratory equipment is emphasized and the possibility of skin irritation as a
marker for exposure is also pointed out. Another interesting series is that reported by Hine (1969) in which
ten cases of methyl bromide intoxication are reported
following exposure from fumigation in the almond industry.
The case reports imply that acute liver injury may occur
as well as acute hemorrhagic pulmonary edema. Both
reports assess the importance for good respiratory equipment for workers who are handling methyl bromide and
both cases also demonstrate the prolongation of symptoms
which may occur following an acute intoxication.

Treatment: Following removal of all contaminated
clothing, washing the skin with soap and water and flushing the conjunctiva or other mucous membranes, treatment
is directed at preventing acute effects as well as the
chronic neurological symptoms. If pulmonary edema is
present, the usual methods of treating such a syndrome
should be entertained, including oxygen, intermittent
positive pressure and so forth. As a general rule,
since methyl bromide is a central nervous system depress-
ant, further central nervous system drugs should be

avoided if at all possible. In the case of convulsions,
it may be necessary to administer a sedative, usually in
the form of diazapam, by slow intravenous drip or use a
barbiturate by the same route. If the fumigant has been
ingested, it must be removed by gastric intubation,
aspiration and lavage. The stomach can be lavaged with
activated charcoal in sodium chloride. Stomach contents
should be analyzed for the presence of bromide ion.

Major treatment is directed at forcing the excretion
of the bromide ion as quickly as possible. This is best
done by intravenous saline or balanced salt solutions
which contain a diuretic such as furosemide. Careful
attention must be paid to electrolyte balance and particularly the replacement by chloride for the bromide
ion. Treatment should be continued until blood bromide
is under 5 mg% and until the patient is fully alert.
In the event of acute hemorrhagic pulmonary edema, the
intravenous fluids must be administered, if at all,
with extreme caution.

Morgan (1977) has also advised the possibility of
using BAL, especially if it can be administered within
a few minutes of absorption of the methyl bromide.

Again, because of the delay in symptoms, it is advisable to follow patients with exposure for at least
48 hours prior to any discharge.

References

DeJong, R.N. (1944) Methyl bromide poisoning.
    JAMA 125:702-703.

Finken, R.L. and W.O. Robertson (1963) Transplacental
    bromism. Amer J Dis Child 106:224-226.

Hane, F.M. and A. Yates (1938) An analysis of four
    hundred instances of chronic bromide intoxication.
    S Med J 31:667-671.

Hine, C.H. (1969) Methyl bromide poisoning: A review
    of ten cases. J Occup Med 11:1-10.

Jameson, H.D. (1979) EEG signs in methylbromide
    intoxication. Electroencephalogr Clin Neurophysiol
    46:2P-3P.

Kagawa, C.M. and C.G. Van Arman (1960) Bromide and
    chloride excretion with diuretic agents in animals.
    J Pharmacol Exper Therap 129:343-349.

Kantarjian, A.D. and A.S. Shaheen (1963) Methyl bromide
    poisoning with nervous system manifestations
    resembling polyneuropathy. Neurol 13:1054-1057.

Moore, M., T. Sohler and L. Alexander (1940) Bromide
    intoxication. Confinia Neurol 3:1-52.

Morgan, D.P. (1977) Halocarbon and sulfuryl fumigants.
    IN: Recognition and Management of Pesticide Poisonings,
    U.S. Environmental Protection Agency, Washington, DC,
    pp. 47-52.

Pollay, M. (1967) The processes affecting the distri-
    bution of bromide in blood, brain, and cerebrospinal
    fluid. Exper Neurol 17:74-85.

Rathus, E.M. and P.J. Landy (1961) Methyl bromide
    poisoning. Brit J Industr Med 18:53-57.

Rosenblum, I, W.R. Stoll, A.A. Stein, E. Goldberg and
    A. Wohl (1963) Hypercholesteremia after administra-
    tion of bromide. Arch Pathol 75:591-594.

Soremark, R. (1960) The biological half-life of bromide
    ions in human blood. Acta Physiol Scand 50:119-123.

Trethowan, W.H. and T. Pawloff (1962) A clinical and
    experimental study of bromide intoxication with
    special reference to bromureides. Med J Australia
    1:229-232.

Ullberg, S. and R. Soremark (1961) Autoradiographic
    localization of bromide (Br^{82} and Br^{80m}) in the
    gastric mucosa. Gastroenterology 40:109-112.

Verberk, M.M., R. Rooyakkers-Beemster, M. DeVlieger
    and A.G.M. Van Vliet (1979) Bromine in blood, EEG
    and transaminases in methyl bromide workers.
    Brit J Ind Med 36:59-62.

von Oettingen, W.F. (1964) The Halogenated Hydrocarbons
    of Industrial and Toxicological Importance,
    Elsevien Publishing Company, Amsterdam.

11

Miscellaneous Herbicides
and Insecticides

Tetradifon

Tetradifon is an insecticide with a molecular formula of $C_{12}H_6Cl_4O_2S$. The structural formula is as follows:

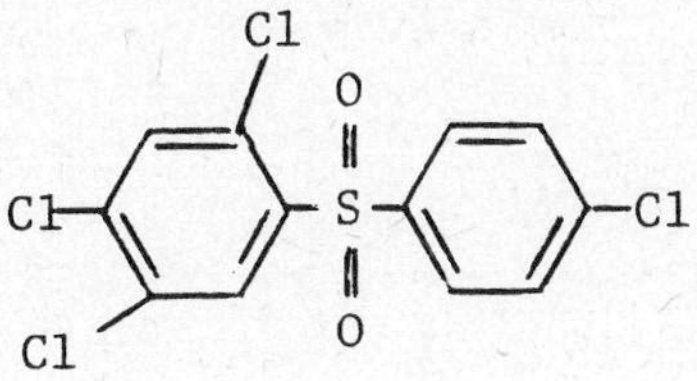

Tetradifon, correctly called tetrachlorodiphenyl sulfone, is an insecticide commonly marketed as Tedion, Mition and Duphar.

The chemical is a colorless crystalline solid with a melting point of 148°C and a density of 2.4×10^{-10} mm Hg at 20°C. It is moderately soluble in water at 0.02 grams per 100 grams and is very soluble in aliphatic and aeromatic hydrocarbons such as CCl_4, methyl acetate, benzene, toluene, xylene and dioxine. It is insoluble in alcohols.

The chemical is generally manufactured by a reaction between trichlorobenzenesulfonyl chloride and chlorobenzene. It is recommended for application to vegetables, ornamentals and nursery stock and has been permitted for use on food for human consumption. The chemical is fairly resistant to acids and alkalies and therefore is compatible with a variety of other pesticides. Chemical analysis for residue is generally through the method of gas spectrochromatography.

Although considered among the less dangerous pesticides, when heated it does emit highly toxic fumes of chlorides and sulfur oxide.

In experimental animals, the chemical has an oral LD_{50} in rats of 566 mg/kg. In dogs, the oral LD_{50} exceeds 2 g/kg.

Rats fed a diet containing 500 ppm of tetradifon for two months suffered no ill effects. Offspring of rats fed 1000 ppm for two months showed no teratogenic changes. When given to rats at 1500 ppm over long periods of time, evidence of hepatotoxicity was seen as a fatty infiltration. Dermal application can cause mild burns of the skin and in the eye.

There have been no reported cases of human intoxication from this chemical in spite of its fairly wide use. Analysis for the chemical in human tissue would be best performed through the method of thin-layer chromatography or gas chromatography.

Glyphosate

Glyphosate, chemically N-(phosphonomethyl)glycine, is commonly marketed under the tradename of Roundup. The chemical is quite new and scientific literature is not yet available although considerably toxicity material has been developed by the parent company.

The rabbit acute oral toxicity study shows an LD_{50} of 3.8 g/kg. A 90 day rat feeding study showed a no observable effect level (NOEL) at 2,000 ppm. A 90 day dog feeding study has shown a NOEL at 2,000 ppm. A two generation rabbit teratology study has been performed which was negative at 30 mg/kg/day, which was the highest dosage although the EPA is currently requesting that further teratology studies be performed, particularly on a second mammalian species. A two year rat feeding study has shown a NOEL of 100 ppm and a three generation rat reproduction study has shown a NOEL of 300 ppm. A neurotoxicity study on hens was negative at 7.5 mg/kg. Further work is still required on this chemical in terms of its possible role as a carcinogen as well as a mutagen.

At the present time, the chemical is licensed for use on foods with an allowable daily intake (ADI) of 0.05 mg/kg/day and an allowable food residue of 0.2 ppm. The theoretical maximum measure of contribution is 0.21 mg/day for a 60 kg person, or 7.06% of the ADI.

The chemical is metabolized to aminomethylphosphonic acid.

Propham

Propham, generically called isopropyl carbanilate, is an herbicide which has the molecular formula of $C_{10}H_{13}NO_2$ and the structural formula is as follows:

$$\text{C}_6\text{H}_5-\text{NH}.\overset{\overset{\text{O}}{\|}}{\text{C}}.\text{O}.\text{CH}\begin{array}{l}\diagup\text{CH}_3\\\diagdown\text{CH}_3\end{array}$$

The chemical is also known under the names of Chem Hoe, IPC and Ban-Hoe.

The chemical has a molecular weight of 179.2 and a specific gravity of 1.09 at 30°C. In the pure state it is a light tan solid which melts at 90°C and sublimes very slowly at room temperature. Rather than boiling, it sublimes upon heating and the decomposition temperature is 150°C or higher. The chemical is practically insoluble in water but is soluble in most organic solvents, particularly carbon disulfide, ethyl or isopropyl alcohol, acetone, benzene and xylene.

The chemical is used as both a pre-emergence and post-emergence broad spectrum herbicide. The formulations are either as an emulsifiable concentrate which is mixed with water at 10-40 gal/acre, or as a granular formulation which involves the binding of 15% propham to a sand-core base. It is generally applied at a rate of one to four pounds per acre. It is loosly bound to soil and water will allow propham to leach or to move.

In experimental animals, propham has an acute oral LD_{50} in rats of 1,000 mg/kg and in mice of 3,000 mg/kg. At 600 mg/kg, the toxic effects include neoplasms. The chemical is believed to act as a two-stage carcinogenesis initiator. In relatively long-term studies, albino rats and beagle dogs fed propham over 90 days at dietary levels of 200 and 2,000 ppm respectively did not show evidence of toxicity. In birds, acute symptoms, principally of central nervous system signs involving ataxia and changes in gait, developed at small dosages.

The chemical has a biological half-life in rats of five hours. The main route of excretion in mammals appears to be via the urine with a small amount appearing in the stool. After oral administration in rats, 80% appeared in the urine within four days. The chemical was evenly distributed with the highest concentration being found in the kidneys. The chemical is conjugated and then excreted as a glucuronide either in the form of metabolic breakdown products such as hydroxycarbinilate or as a sulfate ester.

The preferred laboratory methods for analysis are thin layer chromatography or gas chromatography.

Barban

Barban is a selective herbicide with the generic name 4-chloro-2-butynyl-N-chloro-barbamoate. It has the molecular formula $C_{11}H_9Cl_2NO_2$ and the structural formula is as follows:

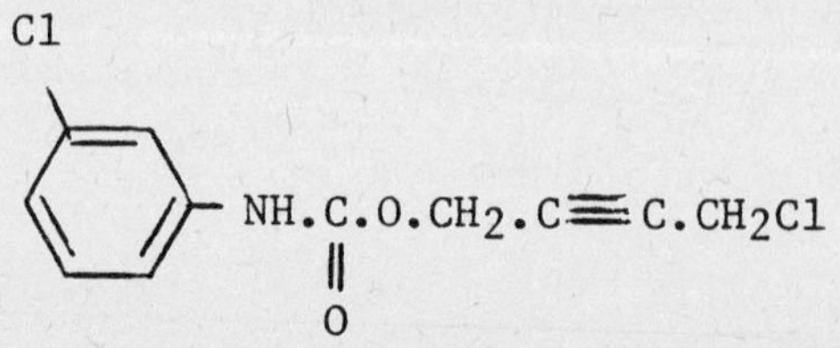

Cl

NH.C.O.CH$_2$.C≡C.CH$_2$Cl
‖
O

The chemical is commonly known under the tradename of Carbyne.

The chemical has a molecular weight of 258.1. The melting point is 75-76°C and the flash point is 81°C. It is a crystalline solid and is colorless in the pure form but the technical material, which is 95% pure, is a pale brown. It is practically insoluble in water (11 ppm) but is readily soluble in some organic solvents such as benzene, N-butylbenzene, ethylenedichloride, toluene and xylene. The chemical stores well but is hydrolyzed easily under both alkaline and acid conditions liberating free chlorine in the former and 3-chloroacrylic acid in the latter.

In the Pacific Northwest, the chemical is used mainly as a selective herbicide for the control of wild oat in wheat. It may also be used in other grain crops as well as vegetables.

Toxicity studies demonstrate an acute LD_{50} in mice of 1,350 mg/kg, in rabbits of 600 mg/kg, in guinea pigs of 240 mg/kg and in rats of 1,350 mg/kg. The inhalation toxicity in rats is 527 mg/kg. The percutaneous LD_{50} in rabbits exceeds 23 g/kg. Goldfish and guppies are susceptible at 1.3 ppm after 96 hours of exposure. Chronic feeding studies in both rats and dogs for periods of 21 months did not demonstrate any abnormal reaction. Barban orally administered to rats is hydroxylated and side chain oxidation occurs leading to the formation of chloro-aniline and the presence of chlorophenols. These are excreted either freely or in a conjugated form. The chemical and its breakdown products are also freely dis-tributed to a variety of tissues in the body.

In the environment, the chemical is usually applied as a post-emergence spray at rates of 0.25-1.0 pounds/acre and the usual carrier is water. It absorbs tightly on soils and microbial breakdown is believed to be fairly rapid with trace amounts present three weeks after appli-cation. The chemical binds tightly to soil and therefore does not leach easily.

Barban is believed to be of low toxicity to man. In spite of its lack of significant skin toxicity or changes, the chemical is highly irritating to human skin and is also a sensitizer to some people. Workers are therefore advised to avoid all types of skin contact by the use of protective plastic clothing and, in addition, to protect the eyes.

There is some suggestion that the chemical may act as a carbamate and therefore cholinesterase levels should be performed on people suspected of an intoxication syndrome, as well as looking for typical symptoms of carbamate intoxication.

Analysis is by several different photometric tech-niques.

Terbutryne

Terbutryne is an herbicide which is of the triazine family. The chemical is manufactured under the name Ingran. It is also known under the names of Prebane and Shortstop.

The chemical has the molecular formula of $C_{10}H_{19}N_5S$ and the structural formula is as follows:

$$
\begin{array}{c}
S-CH_3 \\
| \\
C \\
// \ \backslash \\
N \quad\quad N \\
| \quad\quad || \\
C_2H_5-NH-C \quad\quad C-NH-C(CH_3)_3 \\
\backslash\backslash \quad / \\
N
\end{array}
$$

The chemical has a molecular weight of 221.4 and a melting point of 104°C. It has a low vapor pressure of 9.6×10^{-7} mm Hg. In the pure form, it is a white crystalline solid. It is only slightly soluble in water at 58 ppm but it is quite soluble in a number of organic solvents such as xylene and isopropanol. It is usually manufactured as a wettable powder and then is formulated in water and applied at rates of about 1.2-2.2 lbs/acre for post-emergence application, particularly on wheat.

The chemical is considered to have low toxicological properties. In experimental animals, the acute oral LD_{50} in rats is 2,500 mg/kg and for dust is greater than 8 mg/l of air after four hours exposure. The chemical does have some eye and skin irritating properties although the dermal LD_{50} for rabbits is greater than 10,200 mg/kg. Intoxication signs in experimental animals are either central nervous system with ataxia and convulsions or dyspnea. In long-term feeding studies, beagle dogs receiving 400-1,000 ppm in feed of technical terbutryne over 90 day periods showed no adverse effects. Rats fed terbutryne at dosage levels of 80-10,000 ppm in feed over a period of six months showed effects only at the 10,000 ppm level. A 400 ppm dosage was considered no effect. The results of long-term feeding at high chronic dosage does show growth retardation, slight leukopenia and hepatotoxicity. In extremely severe acute dosages, the principal findings were pulmonary edema and central nervous system edema. Nephrosis and hepatotoxic changes also occurred with high dosages.

In mammals, the chemical can be expected to be conjugated in liver to a glucuronide form and subsequently excreted via the kidney either as a glucuronide metabolite such as triazinyl-s-glucuronide or alkyl-o-glucuronide.

There are no known instances of human toxicity and treatment would be symptomatic including forced emesis or gastric lavage followed by saline laxatives or other supportive therapy.

Laboratory analysis can be performed by gas chromatography.

Metachlor

Metachlor is a pre-emergence herbicide used particularly for the control of broadleaf weeds. The generic name is 2-chloro-2',6'-diethyl-N-(methoxymethyl) acetanilide.

The molecular formula is $C_{14}H_{20}ClNO_2$ and the structural formula is as follows:

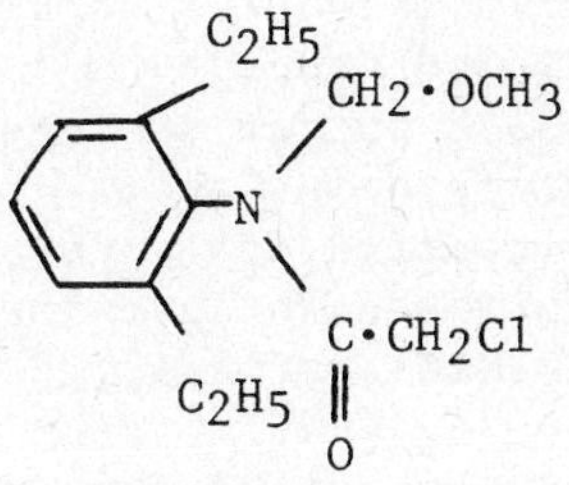

The chemical's molecular weight is 269.77 and the melting point is 40-41°C. Its density is 1.133 at 25°C. It is a cream colored, odorless solid at room temperature. It is soluble in water at 220 ppm. It is quite soluble in ether, acetone, benzene, chloroform, ethanol and ethyl acetate.

In experimental animals, the rat oral LD_{50} is 1200 mg/ kg. The lethal dose in rats via the percutaneous route is greater than 2,000 mg/kg. The chemical is not an irritant to the skin. In rabbits, the percutaneous LD_{50} is 3500 mg/kg.

Although the chemical is of low toxicity, it has a stable residue and has been demonstrated to last some 10-12 weeks after application.

The chemical is considered essentially non-toxic to mammals and has been given an estimated LD_{50} of 3,000 mg/ kg.

Analysis for residues is performed by gas chromatography.

Dicamba

Dicamba is an auxin herbicide with the generic name 3,6-dichloro-o-anisic acid. It is usually marketed under the name of Banvel. Alternative names include Mediben, Banlen and Dianate. It is also formulated with other chemicals, particularly 2,4-D or MCPA as in Weedmaster or Mondak respectively.

Its major use is to control broadleaf weeds on vegetables or grain crops. The usual carrier is water at rates of 2.5 pounds/acre to 0.5 pounds/acre.

The chemical has a molecular formula of $C_8H_6Cl_2O_3$ and the structural formula is as follows:

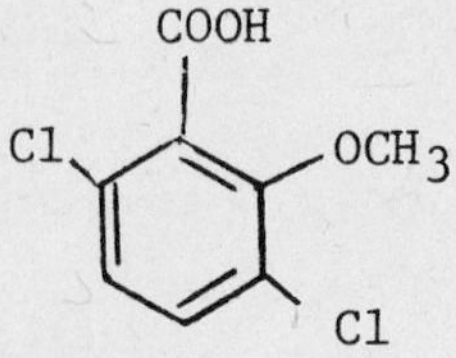

Its molecular weight is 221.05 and its melting point is 114-116°C. In pure form it is a white crystalline solid, however, in technical grade it is a brown crystalline solid. It is fairly stable under most conditions and resistant to oxidation and hydrolysis. It is quite soluble in water at 450 mg/100 ml and the salt is very soluble in water at 38 grams of acid equivalent/100 ml. The usual market form is of the dimethylamine salt which is soluble in water at 72 g/100 ml of water. It is also moderately soluble in ketone, ethanol and xylene. The technical product is about 83-87% pure dicamba. The remainder consists mainly of 3,5-dichloro-2-methoxybenzoic acid and 3,5-dichloro-o-anisic acid.

Toxicity studies in experimental animals have demonstrated an acute LD_{50} in rats of 1,040 mg/kg, in mice of 1,090 mg/kg, in rabbits of 2,000 mg/kg and in guinea pigs of 3,000 mg/kg. Rainbow trout and bluegill showed toxic effects when fed 28 ppm and 23 ppm for 96 hours respectively. Long-term feeding studies with dogs fed for two years at levels of 100 ppm showed no effects either by measures such as weight or by microscopic examination of tissues. Chronic toxicity studies indicate that hepatic necrosis may occur after prolonged ingestion at levels of about 250-400 ppm in the diet. The chemical has been demonstrated to be a mild irritant to the skin of rabbits.

Metabolism studies have shown that when the chemical is given to cows, 73% is eliminated unchanged and 20% is eliminated as a glucuronide conjugate. Therefore, the chemical is partially detoxified by the liver. Given to rats, tissue clearance has been rapid and urine excretion was 96% of the given dose after 24 hours.

In the environment, the chemical is broken down mainly through microbial action. The major metabolic products are either a dichlorobenzoic acid or 3,6-dichlorosalicylic acid. The chemical moves easily through soil. Under conditions which favor biodegradation, i.e. moist conditions, the half-life is about 14 days.

In humans, symptoms which might be expected, although not reported, would involve the liver as the primary site of toxic action. Since the chemical is considered an irritant, every attempt should be made to wash it off with soap and water. Routine first aid would include the use of Syrup of Ipecac or possibly even lavage. Removal of the chemical may be enhanced with the use of a charcoal slurry followed by the use of a saline cathartic.

The principal analytic method for study is via gas chromatography.

Appendix

Alphabetical List of Chemicals in Part II

Index

303